Adventures in Immortality

Adventures
in
Immortality

by George Gallup, Jr.
with William Proctor

McGRAW-HILL BOOK COMPANY
New York   St. Louis   San Francisco
Toronto   Hamburg   Mexico

1 2 3 4 5 6 7 8 9 D O D O 8 7 6 5 4 3 2

ISBN 0-07-022754-3

LIBRARY OF CONGRESS CATALOGING IN PUBLICATION DATA

Gallup, George, 1930–
  Adventures in immortality.
  1. Future life.   2. Death, Apparent.
I. Proctor, William.   II. Title.
BL535.G254   129   81–23638
ISBN 0–07–022754–3   AACR2

Book design by Roberta Rezk

Contents

1

Introduction to
the Adventure

PERHAPS THE MOST provocative question of all time
is, "Does a life exist beyond death?"

This is the basic question that has highlighted
the spiritual speculations of mankind since the dawn
of history. The earliest artists and craftsmen often
made life after death a subject of their cave drawings
or their pottery decorations. Every major religion
has explored the possible landscape of an afterlife.
And in our own day, scientific and quasi-scientific
tools have been employed to study strange and paranormal phenomena which many think may have
some relationship to a life beyond death.

Because of the pressing nature of this topic, I
decided several years ago to turn the full resources
of the Gallup Poll toward an exploration of the afterlife. For about a year and a half, from early 1980
until September 1981, our organization conducted
a series of national surveys probing the attitudes and
beliefs that Americans eighteen and older hold about
immortality.

Using a scientifically selected sampling of people,
we asked, in face-to-face interviews, a number of

1

key questions about heaven, hell and other aspects of life after death. Then, we correlated the responses with a variety of personal data, such as each individual's religious, educational and geographical background.

A special focus of this study has been the involvement of Americans in "near-death" or "verge-of-death" experiences. This aspect of our investigation required in-depth questionnaires calling for open-ended, detailed descriptions of any sort of unusual or "mystical" encounter people may have had when they were at death's door.

In conjunction with this special focus, we conducted two small-scale but statistically representative surveys of national leaders in the fields of science and medicine. The results of these two surveys will be referred to throughout the book, and in accordance with our usual reporting methods, the responses of the scientists and physicians, as of the other respondents, will be quoted anonymously.

Taken together, this series of polls, the specifics of which are given in the Appendix, and other studies we've conducted represent the most comprehensive national survey on beliefs about and experiences with the afterlife and near-death encounters that has ever been undertaken.

Why does this particular topic warrant our special attention? Or, to put it in a more historical context, why has there been such a continuing fascination with the afterlife?

For one thing, we are always drawn inexorably to an investigation of the unknown. But there are darker forces that drive us to ponder the question of immortality. Ernest Becker, the late Pulitzer Prize-winning author of *The Denial of Death* indicated that at the bottom of all our phobias and neuroses lies a fear of death. We're frightened of what may happen to us *at* death—whether the experience will be painful or dehumanizing in some way. But even more disturbing, we're afraid of what may or may not come *after* death. Hence, the ultimate question, "Does a life exist beyond death?"

2

I have asked this question of the American people several times in the past, and the responses are always fairly consistent. In our surveys conducted specifically for this book, about a quarter of our adult population answered "no," there is no life after death. But many more, a full two-thirds of all adult Americans, or about 100 million people, responded with a resounding "yes," and they seem to be part of an ongoing majority throughout history.

But such opinions, while they may be of interest for many reasons, are only part of the story that has been unfolding in recent years about the afterlife. A much more dramatic field of investigation has involved those people who say they have had a close call with death or some other traumatic experience that may have ushered them temporarily into a supernatural realm. Our special national surveys of these reported direct encounters with immortality were followed up by in-depth interviews. We have also sought analyses of our findings by physical scientists, social scientists, theologians and other experts.

The results of all this research don't by any means constitute what might be considered proof of immortality or the afterlife. But of course our purpose hasn't been to provide such proof. Rather, our focus has been upon gathering information in as objective a way as possible, and then letting that information speak for itself. In some cases, our findings confirm studies that have gone before. But we have also discovered new information and have come up with revelations that run counter to previous investigations.

In the following pages, we explore near-death experiences in detail. The Gallup Poll did not try to distinguish between a mystical experience caused by a change in the brain's chemistry and an experience that would best be explained as a revelation of God. Nor did we attempt to learn whether the near-death events that triggered mystical incidents involved what scientists today call brain death (or total cessation of brain wave activity) or merely a close   3 call with death where bodily functions were still operating.

The responses we received often indicated the type of medical phenomenon in question. But the average persons we talked to, who underwent such things as traumatic operations or near drowning, weren't usually in a position to evaluate the precise medical implications of their experience. However, those responding have often indicated whether they had high fevers, were on strong medication, were anesthetized, were drowning or were suffering from carbon monoxide poisoning. These physical symptoms and outside pressures and influences are important in aiding physicians and scientists as they try to distinguish between experiences that are explainable scientifically, and those that are not.

Therefore, we consulted experts in various specialized fields for their thoughts and interpretations of our data. Our surveys and in-depth interviews were designed to provide enough detailed information to give those experts a sufficient data base for their analysis.

Although the main focus of this book will be upon the nature and meaning of the near-death or verge-of-death experience, the discussion will be set against a backdrop of surveys and interviews that reflect many other facets of the American adventure in immortality. We'll consider the broad cultural assumptions and beliefs Americans have about heaven and hell. Also, there will be references to dreams, visions and other phenomena that may provide some elucidation—or at least provoke deeper thinking— about the possible landscape of the afterlife.

2

The Entrances
to Eternity

THERE IS ONE CERTAIN entrance to eternity and that's the permanent termination of life that we call death. But this particular path to the hereafter isn't able to shed much light on our quest during our lifetimes for information about immortality.

Now, even as I make this statement, I'm acutely aware of such accounts as the biblical narratives of ordinary people who died and returned to life. One of the most famous incidents concerns Jesus' friend Lazarus, who, the Gospel of John says, was dead for several days before Jesus called him out of the grave. Unfortunately, though, Lazarus didn't describe what he saw or did during that period in the netherworld—and philosophers like L. N. Andreev have bemoaned this lack of information.

"Why dost thou not tell us what happened in the beyond?" Andreev wrote. "For three days had he been dead. Thrice had the sun risen and set, but he had been dead; children had played, streams had murmured over pebbles, the wayfarer had stirred up the hot dust in the highroad . . . but he had been dead. And now he was among them; he touched them, he looked at them . . . looked at them! And through the black discs of his pupils, as through darkened glass, stared the unknowable beyond."

Although we may not have a Lazarus whom we can question today, we have the next best thing—millions of people who have, by prevailing medical definitions, died briefly or who have come close to death. If you project our findings into the national population, about 23 million people have had a verge-of-death or temporary death experience, and of that number about eight million have experienced some sort of mystical encounter along with the death event.

In addition, there are countless others who claim they have caught a glimpse of eternity through dreams, spiritual visions and other abnormal occurrences which often bear a strong resemblance to the reports of near-death and temporary death adventures.

Our studies suggest there are seven possible entrances, or windows, on the afterlife. Any of these entrances are subject to a number of interpretations: There will be those who say they are nothing more than a window on man's own mind or imagination, and not avenues to a separate, supernatural reality. But many more Americans—more than twice as many according to the surveys—believe there *is* something real out there, beyond our three-dimensional universe. And they also say they think that one or more of these entrances lead to an extradimensional realm, a kind of parallel universe that many equate with heaven or hell.

Entrance 1: Physical Accidents. One of the things that most often triggers an unusual, mystical kind of experience is a serious accident, like a near drowning or car wreck. In all of the cases that we have considered, the threat of death was imminent and some sort of injury occurred, even if the person wasn't pronounced medically dead.

6   One 33-year-old service station attendant from Califor-

nia, for example, reported, "I was drowning in a pool. I got tired and I heard a person calling. I was out of my body calling for help. I was floating and feeling happy and content. I watched them pull me out and saw myself."

In this situation, after a brief period of struggle against danger, the person slipped over into a state of acquiescence, where he relaxed and accepted his fate. It was even an enjoyable experience, despite the threat of extinction of his life. And strange things, such as the out-of-body feeling, began to happen to him.

Car accidents are another trigger to a possible other-worldly encounter. One furniture salesman from North Carolina told us, "In the ninth grade, I was hit by a car while crossing the street. I was reported in the newspapers as having been as high as 30 feet in the air. I remember everything being black and then a big, loud, booming voice commanded me, 'Open your eyes!'

"My eyelids were pushed back, as if by fingers opening my eyes, and my arms were pushed down in front of my head, straight down toward the pavement. These reactions were not my reflexes, but God was helping me by moving my arms and eyelids. I hit the pavement and rolled and received minor abrasions, bruises, cuts and stitches. I would have died by diving headlong into the pavement on the top of my head if God had not helped me and wanted me to live."

In this case, the threat of danger may have focused the person's mental faculties in an almost superhuman beam of concentration that helped him react quickly and effectively to avert serious injury and possible death. Or, as he believes, the nearness of death may have opened a window on eternity and paved the way for some sort of supernatural or extradimensional intervention. In any case, his sense of some power beyond himself is a common experience among those who have been in traumatic car accidents.

People have had similar responses to choking on food, 7

carbon monoxide poisoning, and a variety of other physical accidents that threatened life. Something seems to happen—either through the shock of the car impact or the unexpected, ultimate confrontation with danger—which sets off a series of feelings and events that catapult the individual into another level of reality.

Entrance 2: Childbirth. Although childbirth is generally regarded as a relatively safe procedure these days, there is still enough physical stress and danger associated with it to make it one of the most common entrances to eternity we came across in our in-depth interviews.

Here are some of the reports we received:

• A 60-year-old Kentucky housewife: "When my daughter was born, I almost died. I saw a white cloud and I just drifted away into it. It was so peaceful and I was really amazed when the doctor brought me back to life."

• A 38-year old Michigan mother: "After childbirth I went into shock because of the loss of blood, and I could see everything going on in the room, including my own body lying on the table. I could hear everything—it was as though my spirit had left my body and I was looking down on it."

• A 32-year-old Oklahoma housewife: "I suffered a miscarriage with serious results and extreme pain. I saw Jesus and He explained that He also bore extreme pain on the Cross. And although I could not give live birth to my baby, I should rejoice in giving birth in spirit."

• An elderly Philadelphia resident: "After the birth of my daughter, I was pronounced dead. It was as though I died and went to heaven. I heard people talking and praying at the bed. When I got to heaven, it was like a cloud, and an angel told me to ask the Lord if I could go back and take care of my baby. I walked down on steps of outstretched arms of angels and woke up. I was gone long

8

enough for them to send a telegram and call the under-taker."

There is often a stark contrast between the wrenching fears and anticipation of pain that may precede the near-death event (especially when the person knows a physical test is coming, as in the case of childbirth or slow terminal illness), and the sense of peace that accompanies the actual experience of near death. In every case we've investigated, the anticipation was always worse than the actuality. And in fact, the actuality of confronting and undergoing death frequently seems more pleasant than life itself.

Entrance 3: Hospital Operations and Other Illnesses Involving Drugs or Anesthetics. Whenever the individual underwent a near-death or temporary death event, I've felt it essential to indicate explicitly when anesthetics or drugs were definitely or probably involved. This is, of course, because the drugs themselves may have caused a seemingly supernatural experience. It's interesting to note, however, that there tends to be a certain similarity between the accounts of those who were on drugs and those who were not.

For example, a university student from Wisconsin said, "I had surgery and when I was in the recovery room, I stopped breathing. As they worked on me, I remember feeling like I was not in my body. But I could hear them talking and I felt that I was floating. But it was very black where I was—and I was at peace."

More dramatic, graphic images came to a 50-year-old factory worker from Illinois. After his appendix burst, he was rushed to a hospital, where the doctors pronounced him dead. They left him on the operating table, during which time, he reported, "I saw my [dead] mother. She was in the most beautiful place . . . a real bright light . . . flowers and streams. She told me she was very happy. But   9

she also told me I was to go back home to my family—
that she wasn't ready for me yet. She said that they [my
family] needed me back home. She then bid me good-bye
at a white bridge spanning a stream. I started walking slowly
back. Then I came to, and the nurses and doctors said I
had really died for a time."

A more specifically Christian kind of scene unfolded for
a middle-aged New Jersey housewife who went into the
hospital for an ulcer operation and had to have more than
two-thirds of her stomach removed. She was immediately
put into an intensive care ward for about four days, and
she recalled, "After the first day, I remembered nothing.
Only that a big wind came and took me, still in bed, to a
hilltop, where I preached, sang and played on the piano—
'Let's Just Praise the Lord' was the song.

"I also witnessed [i.e., described her beliefs and faith
experiences] to my family and husband. One day, this beautiful beaming light just glowed on me. I was walking on
what looked like sparkling glass flowers of every kind and
color. The light got closer and closer, and I just knew it
was the Lord Jesus, though I did not see a face, only a
light. And He said, 'You are healed.'

"I went home from the hospital the next morning. They
called me a 'miracle girl' in the hospital. Praise the Lord—
He is my healer."

This woman, a member of an Assemblies of God church,
represents a clearly definable group who perceived a connection between their mystical near-death experience and
their Christian faith. Of those we polled who had a religious
experience involving Christ, 23 percent said they also had
been on the verge of death at some point in their lives.
As a result, it's logical to assume that some definite Christian
content would appear in their descriptions of near-death
incidents.

But it's important to emphasize here that those with
Christian content in their experiences constitute a minority

of those responding. Also, such things as a religious awakening or an indication of religious commitment like church attendance are by no means prerequisites to having a mystical verge-of-death encounter. This type of incident is as likely to happen to those with little or no religious orientation as it is to those who are very religious.

Entrance 4: Sudden Illnesses Outside Hospitals. I distinguish between in-hospital and outside-hospital examples because there seems less likelihood that drugs would play a decisive role in the nonhospital cases.

One elderly woman with a heart condition said, "I had pains in the chest and lay on the davenport and felt like I was fainting. During this time, my [dead] mother came and stood beside me and said, 'Gail, come with me.'

"As she started to walk away, I tried to get up to follow her. But I fell on the floor in a great deal of pain. She continued to walk away and walked *through* the dining room table and the wall and then disappeared. I feel if she had not been there, I would have lost my life."

Another woman, a 36-year-old from California, was pulled back from death by her mother, too—but in this case the parent was alive rather than dead. "While critically ill with pneumonia," she explained, "I had the sensation of my body becoming heavier and seeming to sink down into the mattress, into the springs. Also, I had the feeling that a chill draft was surrounding my body. Yet I seemed to watch all this happen as I—my mind—hovered in midair in the warmth of a soft, comforting light.

"Then, my mother's cries and her warm hand on my forehead seemed to pull my body up out of the cold draft, and suddenly my mind and body came together and I looked up at my mother."

In still another incident, a California social worker said he was suffering from a strep throat infection for which no antibiotics were immediately available. He was treated 11 with heat packs, which were supposed to limit the infection, and was finally taken into a doctor's office for more extensive treatment. While waiting for medical treatment, he "had the sensation of floating two or three feet above the [table]. There were no lights, personages, etc. I awoke days later, alive, after having undergone a tracheotomy."

Even though these out-of-body experiences are by no means the general rule in near-death events, they are cited by a significant number of individuals who have been on the verge of death. In one of our surveys, there is an indication that as many as two million people may have experienced this out-of-body sensation. This figure is not a statistical certainty, however, because in that poll we were dealing with a relatively small sampling of people who reported an out-of-body occurrence.

Entrance 5: Criminal Attacks. A negative, fear-ridden reaction is what you might expect most often from those who are victims of various kinds of criminal attacks. But that's not always the case. Sometimes, these incidents can open the door to a mystical encounter quite similar to those experienced by people involved with accidents or illnesses.

For example, one young New York woman was attacked by a mugger on a Manhattan street, and her purse was stolen. "He came up from behind me, pushed me aside, and took my purse," she explained. "The whole thing really frightened me. But I had felt very close to God that day, and I sensed He was protecting me. I was just thankful that I hadn't been hurt. Then I called the police near the spot where the theft had occurred, and to my amazement, they said they had caught the mugger and recovered my purse.

"The whole incident had me so on edge and excited that I couldn't get to sleep, so I prayed that God would help me sleep. And that's when this strange thing started to happen. I was lying on my bed, and I felt myself being raised outside my body, so that in some way I could now look down on myself. All the weight of the world, the hardships, the worries I had from that incident were gone. There was complete weightlessness, and complete joy. I knew it would be like this when we die, and I didn't want to go back to my body.

"I was in total state of freedom, so that I could move where I wanted in space. But even though I didn't want to go back into my body, I knew I had to. I knew I had experienced a blessing from God for a short time, and now He was saying to me, 'You have to go back.' "

It seems particularly unusual that being the victim of a crime would trigger an experience like this, and it may be that this mystical reaction could only happen if the individual happens to be immersed in a strong inner faith when the attack occurs. But the similarity to the more common near-death accounts is striking, and there probably is some relationship between them. Whenever a crime occurs against a person, there is a sense of having been personally violated. And if the attack is *immediately* personal, as with a mugging, the sense of threat to one's personal safety or even one's life may be enough to stimulate what happens with a bad car wreck, near drowning, traumatic childbirth, or serious illness.

Entrance 6: The Deathbed. There are certain happenings surrounding deathbed scenes that survivors have witnessed firsthand, and these events add to our growing body of information about the other side of death.

A son reported that his mother, in the moments immediately before she died, looked upward and said, "Oh, it's so beautiful!"

In another case a woman who was in the last seconds of life looked up and in the presence of witnesses said, "There's Bill," and then she passed away. As it happened, 13

Bill was her brother and he had died just the week before—but she had never been informed about his death.

One of the best-known people who has witnessed a deathbed encounter with eternity is the evangelist Billy Graham. On the day that his grandmother died, he was sitting by her side in a dark room, when suddenly the room seemed to glow with some sort of light. His grandmother sat up in bed, even though she had been too weak to do so earlier, and said, "I see Jesus. He has His Hand outstretched toward me."

Then she said she saw her dead husband Ben, who had lost a leg and eye in the Civil War. "There is Ben," she said. "And he has both of his eyes and both of his legs!" And then, according to Graham, his grandmother died and the room once again became dark.

There is a correlation between what the witnesses to deathbed scenes report and what those involved in near-death events claim to experience. Our findings suggest that as many as eight million Americans, or about one-third of those who have been involved in near-death occurrences, may have felt the presence of some being or otherwise have had a positive, otherwordly experience. Many of those reporting deathbed encounters are describing something quite similar.

Of course, these reports may all be just a form of wish fulfillment, or a projection into death or the near-death event of what we *want* to occur after this life. In this regard, our Gallup surveys do reveal that what people are experiencing in deathbed and near-death encounters correlates rather closely with what Americans in general say they believe heaven will be like.

More than half of the nationwide sample we polled said they believe heaven will be peaceful; those in the afterlife will be happy; they will be in the presence of God or Jesus Christ; and there will be an all-pervasive love between people in heaven. Also, 42 percent said they think they will

14

see friends, relatives or spouses after they die; 14 percent believe those in heaven will have human form; and nearly 21 percent expect that those in heaven will be recognizable as the same person as on earth.

As you can see, these expectations about heaven in the minds of the general population agree with what many who have undergone mystical encounters say they actually experienced. What may be the connection between the general public beliefs and the near-death reports? It may be that the accounts of close brushes with death are actual evidence to reinforce the general convictions about the supernatural.

On the other hand, the supernatural may not be involved at all. It may be that the average person simply has certain thought patterns and beliefs about immortality that surface during stressful, traumatic incidents and cause him to believe certain things that actually exist only in his mind.

Various psychologists and physicians we have talked to suggest that certain dormant mechanisms in the body and mind may come into play during times of danger and physical shock to prepare us to deal more effectively with serious injury or even death. If such is the case, then it may be better to resort to psychological rather than supernatural explanations to interpret the mystical near-death and death-bed accounts.

But before we jump to any conclusions about the meaning of the near-death experiences, let's explore in more detail some of the possible entrances to eternity that they may open.

Entrance 7: Religious Visions, Dreams, Premonitions and Other Spiritual Experiences. This final entrance to eternity is somewhat different from the others because it doesn't necessarily depend on physical pressures or stresses. But I've included it as one of our entrances for a couple of reasons.

15

In the first place, some of our respondents in the surveys on near-death incidents mention dreams and premonitions as decisive experiences which were present at those times when serious danger threatened them. Secondly, there are huge numbers of people who report in other Gallup polls that they have had special kinds of religious experiences, and these experiences are often characterized by mystical happenings similar to the near-death reports.

For example, a middle-aged woman from Texas said that as she was driving down a mountain and rounded a curve in the road, "I looked up to see a fast-traveling train coming out of the trees. Even though I wanted badly to slam on the brakes, I knew that there was no way to avoid hitting or being hit. So I screamed, 'What should I do?'

"A voice as clear as I have ever heard said, 'Put on the gas!'

"Going against my own will, I tried to beat the train— and I was hit at the back door of the car but never got knocked off the highway and came to a stop on the shoulder of the road. As I opened my eyes, I believed surely I was about to meet my Creator. But I felt surprise, then disappointment, then happiness [to see that I was alive and unhurt]. Nearby workers said that if I had put on the brakes, the train would [have hit me broadside and] dragged the car far down the tracks."

In this case, the person was in great danger and came near death but was uninjured as a result of the incident. She felt that the near disaster brought her into touch with an extranormal reality that in effect warned her and gave her specific directions that saved her life.

In addition to a sense of extradimensional communication triggered by a dangerous situation that doesn't lead to injury, some people report communication through premonitions well before a crisis occurs. One Massachusetts salesman said, "While praying at bedtime, I had a strong visual assurance. A car going around a sharp right-hand curve crashed end over end off an embankment. Then, the palm of a hand was raised in front of me, as if in a warning to stop. Several months later, I was in an accident where a young man died. The happening (including my stopping at the right moment) was exactly as in the vision."

Our surveys have also shown that nearly one-third of all Americans—or about 47 million people—have had what they call a religious or mystical experience. Of this group, about 15 million report an otherworldly feeling of union with a divine being. They describe such things as special communications from deceased people or divine beings, visions of unusual lights, and out-of-body experiences. For instance, one said, "I was reading the Bible one night and couldn't sleep. A vision appeared to me. I was frozen and motionless. I saw an unusual light that wasn't there—but was. There was a great awareness of someone else being in that room with me."

In another case, a young man felt a deep sense of God's presence late one night just before he went to bed. After he climbed into bed, the sense of the supernatural continued to be so intense that his body seemed to become weightless and to rise slightly off his bed.

As we examine reports like these in more detail we find that the mystical feelings that accompany near-death experiences and the spiritual awakenings that occur apart from near-death tend to complement and perhaps even explain one another.

But up to this point, we've been discussing mostly the gateways, the thresholds that lead to a more complex and exciting realm beyond. Now, let's step through the door and see what a few of the nearly eight million people, who have had mystical near-death experiences, report about life on the other side.

3

The Search for Paradise

HUMAN BEINGS HAVE ALWAYS been deeply concerned about what positive experiences and benefits may await them after they die. They have speculated extensively on the possible enjoyable aspects of the afterlife, and they have watched for—and claimed to receive—special revelations from the divine realm on the nature of immortality.

Paradise, however, is an elusive concept in any culture, as can be seen from the variety of ideas about the afterlife that have sprung up in the world's many religions. Indeed, what many western peoples call heaven is a place or concept that has captured the imagination of human beings throughout the world since ancient times.

But is there any correlation between this age-old search for paradise and our recent findings about near-death experiences?

To understand as far as possible what happened to those who have been near death or have actually died medically and then returned to tell about it, it is important to know something about certain historically established spiritual categories and religious beliefs.

19

The reason this information is important is twofold: 1) In the first place, arguments have been made that near-death reports are merely dreamlike figments of the individual's imagination, or perhaps wish fulfillments of deeply held personal desires. To determine whether there is any basis for this contention, it's necessary to see whether or not there is any correlation or divergence between generally held religious beliefs and the description of the near-death accounts. 2) Secondly, even if the near-death accounts are couched mainly in terms of known theology, they may still reflect a genuine encounter with the supernatural. Why should this be? Because it would be natural to expect that the events would be presented in some sort of known or traditional terminology—probably the terminology of popular religion. So the more we understand about popular contemporary religious beliefs, the better equipped we'll be to evaluate and ferret out the essence of the near-death encounters.

The kinds of popular religious beliefs that would affect the way people express their unusual, mystical experiences, would likely arise from two main sources: 1) traditional religious theology, which has sifted down into the thinking of the average person on the street; and 2) popular notions about what the afterlife may be like, notions that can best be identified through national population surveys.

In this chapter, then, we'll touch on some of the sources of traditional theology that may have a bearing on the thinking of those reporting positive, enjoyable near-death experiences. Then, we'll go into these religious notions in more detail in later chapters and also discuss some surveys we've done to show general public beliefs about the afterlife.

Most major religions throughout history have affirmed a belief in a special dwelling place for God or the gods—a realm where some select, blessed humans may also be granted admittance. This transcendent spiritual place or dimension has gone under a variety of names and has pos-

20

sessed a multitude of special characteristics, depending on which set of religious beliefs happen to be providing the answers.

In ancient Greece, poets like Homer gave the name Elysium to the most pleasant of these supernatural realms. Elysium was a pretty meadow on the banks of the river Oceanus at the western edge of the earth. Heroes like Menelaus and others favored by the chief god Zeus were allowed to go there without dying, and they lived in this spot through the rest of eternity in total happiness. The climate was perfect, with no storms or blizzards and they had every imaginable good fruit and drink to consume. Some of the later Greek writers placed Elysium inside the earth, but it remained the abode of those who are blessed by the gods.

Islam offers a picture of heaven somewhat like that accepted by the Greeks, with a paradise full of sensual pleasures, rivers of pure water, opulent mansions manned by obsequious servants, and all the good food that those admitted might want to eat.

Here is a selection of passages from the Koran, which have been compiled in Robert Hume's *The World's Living Religions:* "Verily, the pious shall be in gardens and pleasure, enjoying what their Lord has given them; for their Lord will save them from the torment of hell. 'Eat and drink with good digestion, for that which ye have done,' reclining on couches in rows. And We will wed them to large-eyed maids. . . . And We will extend to them fruit and flesh such as they like. . . . In gardens of pleasure . . . and gold-weft couches. . . . Around them shall go eternal youths, with goblets and ewers and a cup of flowing wine. No headaches shall they feel therefrom, nor shall their wits be dimmed! And fruits such as they deem the best, and flesh of fowl as they desire, and bright and large-eyed maids like hidden pearls, a reward for that which they have done."

The afterlife of Islam is also populated by a host of super- 21 natural beings, including the eight angels who support the throne of Allah (the one God), the 19 angels who guard hell, and the archangel Gabriel. There are also jinn, or genii, who are spirits between angels and human beings. They may be good or evil, but one of them is the worst of all, the devil, called in the Koran *Shaitin* (from the Hebrew *Satan*).

Eastern religions like Hinduism and Buddhism tend toward a more nebulous notion of the positive side of the afterlife—an eventual merging of human individuality into the cosmos for human souls who make it to the pinnacle of perfection after numerous incarnations.

Comparative religions expert Huston Smith of the Massachusetts Institute of Technology says that in Buddhism, nirvana, the ultimate possibility in the afterlife, "is the highest destiny of the human spirit and its literal meaning is extinction." But he also points out in his *The Religions of Man*, "It does not follow that what is left will be nothing. Negatively, nirvana is the state in which the faggots of private desire have been completely consumed and everything that restricts the boundless life has died. Affirmatively it is that boundless life itself. Buddha parried every request for a positive description of the condition, insisting that it was 'incomprehensible, indescribable, inconceivable, unutterable. . . .'"

So even in the abstract concepts of the East, the positive dimension of immortality is the quintessence of all that is positive about reality.

In North America, there is a long and amazingly consistent set of traditions about the destination of the blessed after death. Before the white settlers ever arrived, the American Indian had developed a rather detailed picture of the happy hunting ground. In that ideal afterlife, the souls of dead warriors and great hunters continued tracking and killing plentiful game and feasting to their hearts' content with the supernatural sky people through all eternity.

The personal theology of the Europeans who took over the land from the Indians didn't focus on hunting game in the afterlife. For their culture, however, the picture they painted of heaven as an abode for the blessed was just as idyllic.

Relying on the Scriptures and traditions of their Judeo-Christian heritage, many of them believed in the biblical picture of heaven as the home of God and His entourage of attending angels. Depending on their individual theological convictions, they also thought of heaven as the permanent abiding place of those who had either lived a good life, accepted Jesus Christ as their Savior, belonged to a certain church, been "elected" by God for salvation, or some combination of these qualifications.

But the precise idea that any given individual might have had about heaven could get much more complicated. Because heaven, by definition, is a realm beyond our three-dimensional reality, it has never been quite possible to wrap the human mind or human language completely around the concept. The ancient Hebrews and their later rabbinical interpreters certainly tried to come up with some precise definitions, but in the end, their attempts are more suggestive than definitive.

For example, the Old Testament and related interpretive literature variously refer to heaven as having windows; being a garment in which God wraps Himself; including a metal strip which God polishes with His breath; containing storehouses and bottles which contain the winds and rains; and being situated on pillars.

Even more intriguing is the idea that developed among the Hebrews and continued to some extent into Christian thinking that heaven was divided into several layers or levels—perhaps as many as seven heavens. In support of this idea is the fact that the most common Hebrew word (*shamayim*) and Greek word (*ouranos*) for heaven were used in the plural (*heavens*). Also, there are references in the   23

New Testament to what seem to be special locations in heaven, such as "Abraham's bosom" (Luke 16:22) and "Paradise" (Luke 23:43).

Finally, perhaps the most specific biblical reference to more than one heaven is Paul's indication in 2 Corinthians 12:2 that he was at one point "caught up to the third heaven." Both Jewish and Arabic folklore affirm the notion we've already mentioned that there are a total of seven heavens.

Christians and Jews in the United States who believe in the existence of heaven and who are searching with varying degrees of intensity to grasp a clearer picture of the nebulous notion of paradise have been influenced to one degree or another by these theological concepts and traditions. It's been quite common, for example, for us to hear in our surveys that a person believes in certain stages or levels in heaven. And more than once there has been a reference to religious terms like paradise. But there are also a great many more long-standing religious beliefs that have shaped American ideas of heaven.

For example, some readily available biblical and popular theological sources suggest that heaven has such characteristics as mansions where the blessed live; streets of gold; special kinds of angels like cherubim and seraphim; brilliant light; a palpable atmosphere of love; access to complete intellectual and spiritual knowledge; and the companionship of loved ones and other godly people who have already passed on to the next life.

Also, in the Christian tradition, those deceased humans who have made it to heaven acquire special celestial bodies which can do extraordinary things: They move through solid objects; exist without food or drink and without fear of disease; and reflect the blindingly brilliant light that emanates from God's presence.

With this background in mind, let's now turn to some of the actual experiences that the people we've talked with around the country have had. Then, we'll consider whether these contemporary occurrences are consistent with, and perhaps have been influenced by, traditional notions of heaven or whether we may be dealing, at least in part, with something that is completely new and unknown.

First of all, you'll notice as we proceed with descriptions of verge-of-death experiences that the language used by the individuals involved in them is sometimes taken straight out of the terminology of traditional theology. For example, references to angels or some all-powerful being identified with Christ recur periodically.

But it's important to avoid an automatic assumption that just because this religious terminology is employed, the experiences themselves must simply be a projection of the individual's personal beliefs and religious background, and hence invalid. Remember: If we really are dealing with some sort of supernatural realm in these accounts, human words and concepts will, by definition, be inadequate to convey all of what has been seen, felt and experienced.

To put this in more scientific, or at least quasi-scientific form, you might say we are relatively limited three-dimensional creatures who are incapable of describing sights and events that are multidimensional. The afterlife, in other words, may be in effect what some scientists describe as a parallel universe, which could overlap in part with ours, but which also goes far beyond in ways our senses can't comprehend and our minds and voices can't communicate.

Now, let's take a closer look at what happens at the moment that a person moves from our known, three-dimensional existence into the strange world of the near-death adventure. As we have seen in the previous chapter's examination of the seven entrances to eternity, there is almost always some sort of physical or emotional trauma that jars the individual out of his present conscious environment into another. This may involve a physical injury; a close brush with death such as a near drowning; a threat to personal safety, as with a mugging; or some similar occurrence.

After such a crisis takes place, some people—according to our surveys, a minority of about 35 percent of those with a near-death encounter—find themselves catapulted into another dimension of reality or consciousness.

It's important to note at this point that a substantial number of scientists we've polled in a special survey believe that there's not much to the idea that a person can get a taste of immortality through a near-death incident. In fact, only 16 percent of the scientists we polled said they even believe in life after death (in contrast to 67 percent of the entire American population). And an even smaller number, eight percent, said they believe in heaven (as opposed to 71 percent of the American people at large).

One of the scientists we talked to, an endocrinologist who is a self-described agnostic and firm nonbeliever in both the afterlife and heaven, expressed his views on the near-death issue this way:

"If anyone almost dies, i.e., is resuscitated, then he or she was never dead or near it. An altered state [of mind]? Sure! And one which could produce strange hallucinations conditioned by previous experience and culture. This does not, however, in any way constitute a valid glimpse into a life beyond."

There are, of course, many other people—including many scientists, as we'll see later—who disagree with this viewpoint. But it's important to keep skeptical attitudes like these in mind because there is no definitive proof, one way or the other, about what near-death experiences really mean.

So, whatever the ultimate import of the strange experiences that sometimes follow near-death or temporary death incidents or related traumas, it's clear that something out of the ordinary occurs and the adventure begins with what

I call the vestibule effect. In other words, the individual is beset by a definite sensation that he or she has moved from an ordinary, three-dimensional reality into another dimension, where the usual laws of time and space don't apply.

But even though the person has entered a different sort of consciousness, he or she still participates in some way in the old earthly realm of time and space—hence, the use of the term "vestibule," which is the passage or room just beyond the front door, but before you enter into the main part of the house. These people are in a new reality or consciousness to some degree, but they're not completely in. The front door is still open, so that they can often see or hear what's going on in the region from which they've just departed. But now, instead of being participants in the old life, they've become detached observers who are about to turn their backs on the doorway through which they've just passed and embark on a totally new adventure into the unknown.

This sense of detachment and being able to observe the limited earthly realm from a superior vantage point is often accompanied by an out-of-body feeling and a tremendous sense of mental clarity in watching what's going on among those who are still living.

For example, one 28-year-old Indiana woman reported to us that she and her father were working on her car in a garage while the car was running. The carbon monoxide fumes finally got to her and she passed out, but even though she was in one sense unconscious, in another way she was more perceptive and acutely aware of her surroundings than she had ever been.

She said, "I didn't make it to the door—Dad said he dragged me outside. My experience began here. I was approximately four to five feet above my body looking down at myself lying on the ground, with my father at my head trying to get me up on my feet. My mother and baby sister (then about 16) were both at my right side crying. Mom said, 'Breathe, Jeanne, breathe!' And my sister cried, 'Please don't die. Don't you dare die!' (You see, my husband had just died a month prior in an accident.)

"Mom kept pressing my chest to make me breathe. While looking and watching, I at first didn't realize what was happening—why they were crying—because I felt fine. No pain, just joy."

In many other near-death cases, there has been a similar initial interaction between the old, everyday realm of reality and the new one that the person is experiencing. Then, the old life fades away and the person becomes totally immersed in the new, until he or she is jerked back finally into the here and now.

This is the sort of thing that happened to the young Indiana widow we've been considering. After observing her relatives working on her lifeless body, she turned away from them, into the joy she was sensing: "I then looked around to find some explanation. I was not afraid but only concerned about my parents and my sister."

Then, she began to move back to the three-dimensional world again: "The next awareness was I was following my mom, dad and sister, walking along the side of the house, kind of half dragging, half walking. I was pretty much on the same level following them—but not walking, though. I was outside of the body again—still feeling okay, no fear or pain, still wondering why everyone was so upset.

"Then, next thing I remember, I was back in my body because I looked at myself and tested my control over my body. Everyone—the rest of my family—asked if I was feeling better. I was conscious but a little dizzy. Eventually, I did go to the emergency room to clear out my lungs."

It's not always obvious in these near-death experiences at what point the transition stage or vestibule effect merges into an awareness more completely fixed in the afterlife, in which the individual is no longer aware of what's going on back on earth. Sometimes, earthly events pop up periodically and other times, there is a smooth movement from ordinary life to vestibule to a total kind of extradimensional experience.

In some respects, the reports we've received have parallels in contemporary speculative metaphysical literature. For example, take the twentieth-century Oxford scholars Charles Williams and C. S. Lewis. In Williams's fictional study *All Hallows' Eve*, which has been described as a supernatural thriller, he introduces us to a young woman, Lester Furnival, who seems in the first few pages to function just like any other ordinary young woman. But as we move further into the book, we discover that she and some of her friends, even though they are observing and in some cases interacting with the world of the living, have recently died.

At one point, for example, Lester sees her former husband Richard walking toward her: "She went after him; he should not evade her. She was almost up to him and she saw him throw out his hands towards her. She caught them; she knew she caught them, for she could see them in her own, but she could not feel them. . . . As if he were a ghost he faded; and with him faded all the pleasant human sounds—feet, voices, bells, engines, wheels—which now she knew that, while she had talked to him, she had again clearly heard."

Williams's deceased humans, just after they have passed away, have bodies that are recognizable and that give their personalities an identity similar to those they had in life. But there are differences: They can't be seen by living beings; they have much more mobility than earthly creatures; and they tend either to get stronger and more powerful than they were when alive or to shrivel and fade away, depending on their ultimate destiny in the afterlife.

C. S. Lewis uses a similar device in his popular book *The Great Divorce*. In the first pages, he pictures a group

29

of rather ordinary-looking and -sounding people waiting for a bus. They're grumbling about the lateness of the driver and otherwise behaving as though everything were business as usual—until the bus leaves the ground and heads up into the clouds. The passengers, who it turns out have just died, can look back and see the earth for a while, but their final destination is a light-filled, luxuriant land, the entrance to which is bordered by a huge cliff.

They learn later that their new land is a kind of peaceful, idyllic, supremely happy "staging area" on the edge of heaven. And they have unknowingly increased so much in size in their trip that the cliff they originally thought was so large is actually no bigger than a blade of grass in their new abode.

These and other theological beliefs and speculations bear some interesting similarities to the concrete reports we've received from those who have undergone near-death incidents. But, as will be seen, the empirical evidence we've gathered also has many distinctive features that go well beyond these accounts.

4

The Extradimensional
Universe

AS THE SEARCH FOR PARADISE has proceeded in the
world's various religions, there has been little concrete data in the past to add to or detract from the
beliefs based on scripture and divine revelation. But
now, all that seems to be changing.

A growing number of researchers have been
gathering and evaluating the accounts of those who
have had strange near-death encounters. And the
preliminary results have been highly suggestive of
some sort of encounter with an extradimensional
realm of reality. Our own extensive survey is the
latest in these studies and is also uncovering some
trends that point toward a super parallel universe
of some sort—but with a few important new twists.

The responses to our national study of those who
have had a close brush with death reveal ten basic
positive experiences that may have some connection
with what we have always described as heaven. Here
is a summary of those experiences with some indications as to the approximate number of people who
were involved in each type of encounter or sensation:

• An out-of-body sensation: 9 percent of adults with a near-death experience, or about two million people

• Visual perception of something going on around them, either in the earthly realm or some other dimension or level of consciousness: 8 percent, or nearly two million people

• Audible sounds of human voices, either on earth or in some other dimension: about 6 percent of adults with a near-death experience, or about one-and-a-half million people

• An overwhelming sense of peace and painlessness: approximately 11 percent, or more than two-and-a-half million adults

• The sight of a single light or several bright lights: about 5 percent of those with a near-death encounter, or more than one million people

• The impression of reviewing or reexamining the individual's past life in a brief, highly compressed period of time: a solid 11 percent of those we polled, or more than two and a half million adults

• A special sensation or feeling, such as being in another world: about 11 percent, or more than 2½ million adult Americans

• A feeling that another being or beings, other than the living humans who had been left behind, were present during the near-death adventure: approximately 8 percent of those involved in a near-death experience, or nearly two million adult Americans

• A sense of the presence of some sort of tunnel: about 3 percent, or slightly more than half a million people

• Premonitions about some event or events that would happen in the future: about 2 percent, or approximately a half million adult Americans.

One interesting conclusion that can be drawn from this overview of the positive near-death experiences we've studied—experiences that may perhaps shed some light on the nature of the enjoyable or positive dimension of the after-life—is that it's hard to draw any broad generalizations. The picture that comes across is much more complex than some of the pat models or conclusions that have been offered in the past.

For example, it's true that we've encountered some people who report a being of light or a tunnel. And when you project our percentage figures into absolute numbers of individuals, the results look impressive indeed.

But when any given set of figures is compared with the total number of individuals who have had a close brush with death—or with those who have had quite different experiences during a near-death incident—then the impact of the tunnel or being of light becomes less significant. In any case, there is such a wide variety of reports, many of which don't overlap with any other sensations and experiences, that it doesn't make much sense to say that it's probable that you'll see a tunnel or special being when death stares you in the face.

Now, to get a more complete picture of these ten heavenly experiences, let's examine each in greater detail, with some concrete examples from our study.

1. The out-of-body sensation. We've already looked at several examples of this phenomenon, but there are some other interesting points related to the subject. Keep in mind that only a small minority of people who have a close brush with death or some similar trauma ever encounter the out-of-body experience.

We know that the out-of-body event, when it takes place, always seems to occur immediately after the physical or emotional trauma that triggers the whole experience. In other words, the person is hit by a car, nearly drowns or whatever, and without delay, he senses he's no longer attached to his body. In addition, the separated aspect of the person still clearly retains the person's identity. In fact, the conscious identity of the person usually seems to reside   33 wholly in the floating "ghost" and to have abandoned entirely the physical body.

Also, the disembodied spirit of the individual possesses the ability to see and hear clearly what's going on around it, and often its vantage point is from above the surrounding events and people. Furthermore, this out-of-body dimension of the personality is permeated by a sense of well-being and is highly mobile—not at all constrained by our usual limits of time and space.

One fascinating account that we came across in our study involved a middle-aged Oklahoma housewife who was in the process of giving birth to her third child. She said, "I was in hard labor from two A.M. until two P.M. I was yelling for a 'C section' just before Daniel was born, but my doctor said, 'Shut up!'

"I wanted to die of shame for yelling. I wanted to die more than anything! At that moment, I just popped out of my body and was about two or three feet above myself and everyone in the room. My doctor said, 'My God! My God!!'

"Someone moved to my side and pounded on my chest. (I wondered why he was hitting my chest.) Daniel was coming out and was handed to a nurse and wrapped in a blanket. I looked up and saw many beings waiting on me but not talking. We all *knew* each other's thoughts. (This was very beautiful.)

"I turned around wondering about my husband and started to go out the door, but only floated through the door and down the hall to where he was standing in a doorway with my eight-year-old daughter. They were fine—I went back to the birth room.

"The 'beings' were waiting on me to decide to stay with them or reenter my body. It was *my* decision! I wanted to stay on the other side, but felt I should stay and raise my baby until he was 11 years old.

"Immediately, I popped back into my body. My boy is

now 13 years old, and I keep finding another project to start or finish before I leave again."

The tremendous detail in this woman's recollection of her experience is one of the distinctive things that sets her account apart from many others. But many of the points she recounted, such as the immediate movement into an out-of-body consciousness and the great mobility and acute perceptive abilities of her spirit, coincide with what other people have told us. Also, she introduces another interesting trait of the disembodied state: the option to return to an earthly existence or remain in the world of the spirit.

This apparent ability to choose to stay in the extradimensional world or to come back is a thread that runs through other near-death accounts. One young nurse we talked to in Minnesota said her husband was given an erroneous dose of medicine in the hospital and later "described seeing his own body in the process of death and said he felt he had the choice to return or not before being medically revived."

Another interesting twist on the out-of-body phenomenon involved a 34-year-old California entrepreneur who recalled a threat to his life that occurred when he was only ten years old.

"I went swimming at a pool in Detroit," he said. "I was tired but took the dare of friends and tried to swim the width of the pool. I became very sleepy and relaxed and then heard someone calling for help. I felt like I was floating. I remember thinking that whoever was calling for help would be embarrassed when they were saved.

"I then realized I was above everything and looking down at the pool and people. There was a warm bright light in front of me. I did not see any people except those below me. As I looked down I saw it was *me* calling for help! I was scared; then the next thing I remember I was lying on the deck of the pool having artificial respiration administered to me."

35

Once again, many of the main features of this account are similar to those in some other near-death experiences, even though the setting and situation are different. One unusual factor in this incident, however, is that the person who nearly drowned not only observed his body below him, but he also saw and heard himself react in fear to the threat of death.

In other words, the person's self was, in a sense, divided into two parts. The one that remained with the physical body was apparently unconscious because the individual doesn't remember being in his body at the time, only observing it in a detached fashion. But at the same time, that self in the body was quite alive and capable of expressing fear by shouting.

The other self seems to have been more closely connected with the person's conscious identity because when he tells the story of what happened to him, he refers to his disembodied self as though that were really he and discusses the self in the body as though it were a separate person. The true continuity in his personality moves from the self in the body before the drowning incident, into the self in the out-of-body state, and finally back into the self in the body when the resuscitation is taking place.

Before we shift to the next type of positive or heavenlike near-death experience, there's one more important point that should be made about this out-of-body thing. As with most strange, extranormal kinds of experiences, the usual categories we have in ordinary language just aren't adequate to describe what has happened.

We can suggest what the incident was like and perhaps even approach the truth or reality of what happened. But ultimately, we always fall short with our words. Only those who have actually undergone an extraordinary occurrence can combine their words with their inner, ineffable impressions of the event to come truly close to an accurate understanding of what happened.

36

This inadequacy of human language comes across regularly in religious literature. For example, it seems fairly clear that Moses had some sort of extraordinary experiences up on Mount Sinai and elsewhere during the Israelites' 40-year trek through the wilderness after their escape from Egypt. Yet when attempts are made in the Scriptures to explain the nature of his encounters, supernatural, anthropomorphic language has to be used because there are no words that can fully capture and express the total experience.

As an illustration of this, look at the account in Exodus 33:18–23. There, Moses asks God, "I pray thee, show me thy glory." And God responds in effect that Moses can't see Him head-on in His complete glory because that would be too much for any human being. But God does say, "Behold, there is a place by me where you shall stand upon the rock; and while my glory passes by I will put you in a cleft of the rock, and I will cover you with my hand until I have passed by; then I will take away my hand, and you shall see my back; but my face shall not be seen."

Almost any Bible scholar would agree that God doesn't have a hand, back or face in the same sense human beings do. But those inadequate words are as close as the writer of Exodus could come to describe what Moses actually did see—and only Moses knew just how insufficient the human terms really were.

Similarly, when we speak of out-of-body states or refer to concepts like conscious spirit and ghost, we're just shading in a part of the reality that those we surveyed encountered.

But as important as the out-of-body experience has been to some people, it's still only one part of the total picture presented by those who have had a strange near-death experience. Now, let's shift our attention to the second major positive aspect of some near-death experiences—the visual perception of certain things happening around the person who is in the midst of an extradimensional adventure.

2. An acute visual perception of surroundings and events during the near-death experience. For some reason, the senses seem to be heightened during some of the near-death incidents. But the strange thing is that much of this "sense" perception seems to take place in a disembodied state, away from the person's eyes and bodily optical equipment. Part of what is seen is related to the mundane events taking place around the person's physical body. But other visual perceptions, if they can really be called visual, are more directly connected with what the person "sees" as part of the landscape of the extradimensional reality.

We've already discussed several incidents involving people who said they floated up above their bodies and then observed in minute detail the things that were going on around them. In a number of cases, the things they saw, including events outside the room where their physical bodies lay, were corroborated later by witnesses who were conscious during their entire experience.

But again, it's important to remember that most people who had strange perceptions during a close brush with death didn't report things quite like this. A more common kind of visual impression may really have been closer to what we define as a dream than something seen with the eyes because of the strange nature of the reports.

For example, one 64-year-old Texas housewife told us she saw "fields and fields of flowers, each petal distinguished" after having a close call with death. It's fairly clear that there was no scene quite like that in the vicinity when she became unconscious.

Another middle-aged woman who was semiconscious after a serious operation said she found herself walking on what looked like "sparkling glass flowers of every kind and color around. . . ."

A third woman, a young artist, said, "I was very sick and on heavy medications. I was hurting very badly that night. I also took a lot of medicine and went to sleep. I felt lighter and lighter.

38

"All I can remember after that is I was in a house. It had many doors and rooms. I kept opening doors and each time my body hurt less. I finally opened a door to the outside. It was beautiful. Very cool on my face and sunny, clear but not too clear. A lot of green.

"A woman said, 'Relax and enjoy.' But I knew soon I would have to make a decision to stay or not. But if I did want to go back, I had to move my body. I went back, and my body was very hard to move. In fact, I saw my husband. He was very upset. He couldn't wake me. He was pushing me. I thought that was enough, so I went back somewhere different. I could hear my husband call me. And I came back [riding on the back of] many smiling animals. Then, I woke up. There is much more to this, but I didn't have enough room [on the questionnaire]. Sorry. But I'm sure if my husband didn't try so hard to wake me, I wouldn't have come back."

It's quite clear, of course, that most or all of this woman's perceptions about where she was and what was going on around her may have been influenced by the drugs she was taking. But at the same time, there are other cases where people refer to such things as a sunny landscape, flowers and streams even though they haven't been involved with medicine or drugs. In fact, we've discovered generally that people may report similar experiences whether they've been on drugs or not. In other words, there is no distinctive kind of account or response that can be tied exclusively to drug ingestion.

Of course, it is true that some of these visual reports may be more characteristic of a dreamlike state than of a clearheaded optical perception. The person may have slipped off into some sort of sleep, and then his subconscious may have begun to draw pictures and scenes in dreams, which he erroneously interpreted to be part of a special kind of near-death adventure.

But we're moving onto very uncertain ground here because no one really knows where a dream may end and a near-death adventure may begin. Nor is it obvious when the entire near-death experience may be nothing more than a dream. Also, some medical research has suggested that there are different kinds of dreams, depending on the person's stage or intensity of sleep.

Shirley Motter Linde and Louis M. Savary, authors of *The Sleep Book,* say that sleep research has shown that people dream exciting, dramatic, fast-moving, and fantasy-laden dreams during REM or rapid-eye-movement sleep (which seems to occur during moderately deep sleep periods). On the other hand, Linde and Savary say, there are other types of dreams that occur outside of the REM sleep pattern, and this type of dreaming sometimes "gives the dreamer a feeling of 'wandering in a no-man's land,' feeling lost or floating. Often he holds conversations with ghostlike characters. One person awakened from a non-REM period said, 'I was walking, or rather floating, along a street, and there was someone floating toward me. I don't know who it was or where I was. I think I asked the person where I was. Gosh, it reminds me of T. S. Eliot's "Little Gidding"— you remember those lines—"In the uncertain hour before the morning, Near the ending of interminable night . . . Between three districts whence the smoke arose I met one walking . . . As if blown towards me." '

"The non-REM dream seems to depict either a world that is strange, gray, shadowy, floating and mysterious— or one characterized by logical reasoning and thinking that makes the dreamer believe he is not asleep and dreaming, but really awake and thinking of things."

Such descriptions of non-REM dreams, which may occur in either deep or light sleep, are reminiscent of some of the reports we've received from those involved in near-death encounters. On the other hand, there are also elements of the more vivid, narrative-oriented REM dreams that suggest elements in the verge-of-death incidents.

One problem with correlating the near-death experience too closely with dreaming, however, is that there is often a definite interaction between the real world and the near-death spirit world, whereas the dream state mostly involves a complete separation from everyday life. Also, even though there is great variety in the descriptions of near-death experiences, there is at the same time enough similarity in the perceptions of many people to justify distinguishing the near-death incidents from the highly individualistic dream state. Thus, even though we have found in our study that there is no single overriding feature that characterizes the near-death mystical occurrence, there do seem to be ten major categories of sensations and experiences. Dreams, on the other hand, tend to deal with a much broader, perhaps even an infinite spectrum of visual perceptions and other experiences.

Sight is not the only sense that may accompany the positive near-death encounter. Sounds of various kinds may also be present.

3. Audible sounds coming from real people talking in the vicinity of the person who is close to death, or from some extradimensional source. We've already examined a number of cases in which the person involved in the close brush with death heard voices from physicians, loved ones or others at his bedside and responded in some way to the audible commands or supplications.

For example, there was the case in which the very sick young California artist came back to the world of the living only because her husband at her side was so insistent in his pleading.

In another similar case, a Florida woman, at the age of 16, said she "had a bad infection in my foot—unknown to my mother. When the pain was unbearable and I felt sick, I told her. She called the doctor, but by that time my body was stiff and in extreme pain.

"I remember the doctor giving me a shot, and my   41

brother and mother crying—and also something about a hospital. While my mother was holding me, I felt a great release from pain and drifting away (could have been the medication). I heard my mother calling me—calling and calling. I did not want to answer. She was insistent. Finally, I did answer (through habit, I guess). Then, everything was the same, except less pain. The doctor said I didn't have to have a spinal tap, that I'd come through. After a few weeks, I was up and fine."

The fact that this person heard the voices of real people in her physical vicinity suggests that she was either in the extradimensional vestibule we've talked about or she was just slipping in and out of a semiconscious state as a result of the trauma and the medication. But there are other incidents that seem to suggest voices that aren't connected with our ordinary three-dimensional reality.

In one such case, a corporate lawyer from Arizona reported, "I had had pneumonia three times in one month but was just out of the hospital. On the way home from work on a very cold, very dark Denver night, a voice said, 'You are to go to Phoenix.'

"I thought someone had spoken to me. I looked about me and saw a young person approaching me. I asked, 'What?'

"But the young person answered, 'I didn't say anything.'

"That scared me and I hurried to my apartment. That evening, I began to think I was a bit crackers. The following evening after a light supper, I went to bed to get the most rest (doctor's orders). I had my TV on.

"Suddenly, the audio faded, the city noise stopped and the light grew soft in my room. I was about to get up when the voice spoke. It was masculine, gentle, baritone: 'Don't worry. You are not losing your mind. You are to go to Phoenix. Put things in order. You *will* go.'

"I felt less pain, at peace and in a few moments the light was harsh, the city sounds crowded in again and the TV audio came up and all was as before.

42

"All but me, that is. In eight months, I had done what was necessary. I departed for Phoenix without much money and no job. Yet all was well."

The experience that triggered this event was somewhat different from many of the other near-death encounters we've considered up to this point. Even though it followed a serious physical problem that could have taken the man's life, the bodily trauma or possible threat to the person's life was more distant than is the case with a near-drowning or devastating auto accident. Still, the presence of an authoritative voice that gives certain directions or makes pleas is a common part of a number of near-death reports and this one, in the midst of a recovery from a serious illness, fits into some of the other accounts that have been told to us.

So the near-death incidents and related mystical encounters may include a sense of separation of body from mind or spirit, the visual perception of something going on in the extradimensional realm, and the sound of familiar or quite unfamiliar voices. But there is also a special set of feelings that seem to pervade the consciousness of many who have a close brush with danger.

4. *An overwhelming sense of peace and painlessness.* One of the most common reports we heard from those who had tasted death and returned was that it was an extremely pleasant experience. Granted, only about 11 percent of those who had a near-death encounter used explicit terms like "peace" and "painlessness." But still, the overall impression conveyed in the descriptions of approximately one-third of those who came close to death was that they felt positive about the incident—and even thoroughly enjoyed it.

For example, one young Wisconsin man who was undergoing serious surgery said, "When I was in the recovery room, I stopped breathing. As they worked on me, I remember feeling like I was not in my body, but I could hear

43

them talking and feeling that I was floating. But it was very black where I was. And I was at peace."

Another man, a 65-year-old Ohio native, said of his heart attack: "It was a very beautiful experience to me, and personally I wish the cardiac team had not brought me back to life—but for my wife and child."

In a similar vein, a 32-year-old self-employed bread salesman from Pennsylvania reported, "I was very sick in the hospital with two infections and then took on a third, a staph infection. I went delirious. At one point, I remember getting a sharp pain going through my whole body which I can't explain. I asked my girlfriend at the time to pass me my rosaries, as if I knew I was going to die and I needed God's help.

"I passed out holding the cross and squeezing her hand real tight, as I was told later. For such a short period I had no pain or anything, just floating lightly. In that short time, God must have told me that He needed me here."

In these and related accounts, the feeling of the individual was that his physical pain had passed, and he had moved into some sort of pleasant, relaxed and often beautiful state or dimension to ride out the crisis.

Some physicians believe that there is a built-in mechanism in the human body that allows us to experience pain and tension up to a point, but then cuts the pressure off and leaves us in a painless and even pleasurable condition. This same sort of mechanism may be operating in the out-of-body accounts, in that when the pain gets too acute, the conscious mind detaches itself in some way from the body and relates to the injured flesh as to an outside object. Some medical experts have speculated that this ability to detach oneself from pain and move into a near-euphoric state is somehow related to the electrical activity in the brain.

In other words, it may be that when the intensity of the pain or the severity of a physical blow or trauma reaches a certain level, the electrical activity in the brain develops, in a sense, a short circuit. This may help the person escape temporarily from the pangs of the injury through a rather pleasant sort of numbness or sense of detachment.

5. The presence of a blindingly bright light or series of lights. A relatively small 5 percent of those who had a near-death encounter said they saw any lights. As a result, this type of experience can't in any way be regarded as typical or normative, despite what some other researchers have suggested.

At the same time, however, this 5 percent may represent as many as one million adult Americans, and that's quite a substantial number of people to have one particular type of experience. Also, in almost every case where it is mentioned, the light becomes a highly important part of the scene that the individual encounters.

For example, one 32-year-old Iowa housewife told us, "I was choking—had sugar in my windpipe. First, I struggled for breath and then suddenly all pain and panic ceased. All was intensely dark and cool. Someone met me, held onto my right elbow and forearm and guided me as we walked or floated down this long hallway.

"It seemed windy, but I couldn't actually feel the wind. Just about then, I began to see the most beautiful, vivid purplish color of radiating light. It was just around a corner, and I couldn't wait to round that corner and see what I knew would be God. I never made that bend because I was revived. There was such an overwhelming feeling of love and brotherhood, such acceptance and total tranquillity. Total well-being. (It's so very hard to describe all this with mere words.) I believe I was met by my grandfather, who had died well over ten years earlier."

The key reference in this woman's account is "the most beautiful, vivid, purplish color of radiating light" which she said she saw.

Sometimes, the light that is reported is "soft and com-   45 forting" and other times it's brilliant and blinding. On occasion, the light is also connected with some sort of being or a group of beings in the extradimensional sphere.

There are many possible explanations, both scientific and theological, for the vision of light perceived by people involved in a close brush with death. Some medical experts, for example, have reported cases of various sensations of light by people who have suffered blows to the head or other severe outside pressures. They speculate that because electrical impulses are involved in brain activity, the outside trauma (or some serious inner stress) may cause the normal function of these electrical charges to go temporarily haywire, with the result that some sections of the brain may get overcharged with electricity. This could result in a perception of light, even though from an external vantage point there is no light. Sometimes, lights may also seem to be exploding in front of the person's eyes when a brain seizure of some sort is occurring.

A related phenomenon is what psychologists and biological scientists call synesthesia. This term refers to an inner or subjective feeling of a particular sensation at the same time that a completely different sense is being stimulated. In other words, the sense of touch might be stimulated by a severe physical blow, and one of the results could be some visual or audible sensation (in addition, perhaps, to the painful sense of touch).

One type of synesthetic sensation that is directly related to the lights we've been talking about is called a photism. A photism is any visual sensation—often including bright, illuminating lights—that may accompany some entirely different and seemingly unrelated sensation.

For example, the philosopher and religious researcher William James referred in his classic *Varieties of Religious Experience* to the possible presence of photisms during many dramatic religious conversion experiences. One of the most famous accounts of this type was that of the Apostle

46

Paul on the road to Damascus. Paul told King Agrippa in Acts 26:13–15: "At midday, O king, I saw on the way a light from heaven, brighter than the sun, shining round me and those who journeyed with me. And when we had all fallen to the ground, I heard a voice saying to me in the Hebrew language, 'Saul, Saul, why do you persecute me?'"

A similar kind of thing happened to the nineteenth-century Christian leader, Charles Finney. He described his own conversion experience this way: "All at once the glory of God shone upon and round about me in a manner almost marvelous. . . . A light perfectly ineffable shone in my soul, that almost prostrated me on the ground. . . . This light seemed like the brightness of the sun in every direction. It was too intense for the eyes. . . . I think I knew something then, by actual experience, of that light that prostrated Paul on the way to Damascus. It was surely a light such as I could not have endured long."

A contemporary scientist-theologian, Kenneth Boa, has discussed these experiences in relation to the photism concept in his book *The Return of the Star of Bethlehem* and has also tied them to the idea of the *Shekinah* glory or presence of God, which is mentioned throughout the Old Testament. The *Shekinah,* by the way, is frequently associated with overpowering visions of light. These include such things as the pillar of fire that accompanied the Israelites during the nights in their wanderings through the wilderness after leaving Egypt, and also the light that caused Moses' face to shine when he came down from one of his periodic chats with God (see Exodus 34:29–35).

The presence of some sort of light during near-death and related experiences smacks strongly of mysticism and nonrationality. But there are other experiences that are much more concrete and tied more clearly to life on earth. One of these is the frequently mentioned experience, "I saw my whole life pass before me in a flash."

47

6. *A fast review or reexamination of the individual's life.* The largest number of those we polled—about 11 percent of those who came close to death, or about 2½ million adult Americans—reported this perception.

One doctor from Maryland told us, "I was traveling by auto at 55 m.p.h. when the car went out of control on a damp blacktop pavement. Steering was of no use, so I just braced myself against the top part of the inside of the car and hoped for the best—as the car spun.

"My life passed quickly through my mind. (The car struck a soft dirt bank backwards, totaling the car, but I suffered no injury. The seat back absorbed the impact.)"

In a slightly different sort of account, a second doctor who responded to our surveys, a professor of medicine, said he "almost drowned. Time passed slowly, and I could leisurely review my life, friends, foes, etc.—all within the space of a few minutes."

A third physician we questioned, a California pathologist, said he was "swept overboard at sea as a young man but survived. Brief, compressed, apparently unrelated events of my life flashed before me."

Finally, a self-employed California man reported, "While under water in a bay off the Philippines, having surfaced three or four times calling for help, I went through a desperate struggle to resurface. This was followed by a sequence of events relating to my life in high quantity, like a fast movie flashing in my eyes. Then, I must have collapsed. The next thing I knew I was lying on the dock with several people around me, and one person attempting to revive me through artificial respiration. I became ill, but within an hour or so, I was fully recovered."

One of the most interesting things about these accounts and others like them is that the individuals felt that somehow they had entered a new time dimension. Many more things passed through their minds in a short period of time than would be possible under normal circumstances. Also, the pictures and thoughts of their past lives were in a

48

sense forced on them—or at least were run through their minds in a rushed sequence over which they had no control.

A similar kind of experience was reported by an ex-convict named Nick Pirovolos, who was suffering from a severe gunshot wound in the head when he was serving time in the Ohio State Penitentiary for armed robbery a number of years ago. In this recent autobiography, *Too Mean to Die*, he said he was in excruciating pain, and the prison doctors weren't entirely sure he would recover. But then one night he felt a comforting presence—which he was certain was the presence of God—and his entire past life began to pass in front of his eyes. It was a kind of mental movie, but one over which he had no control—at least not until the last reel inside his brain had run its course several hours later.

The upshot of Pirovolos's experience was that he underwent a profound spiritual conversion and became a leading prison evangelist. But the nature of his adventure, except for its extreme length, bears many similarities to what others have reported after serious injuries. In particular, his memory of the experience is that it was arduous but ultimately satisfying and beneficial to him. In other words, in his view it was a positive encounter with the supernatural.

The next major heavenlike characteristic we've encountered in our study is rather hard to define and tends to overlap with some of the other concepts. But it's important enough to have been mentioned by 11 percent of those who had near-death experiences, or perhaps nearly three million people.

7. A special sensation or feeling, such as the impression of being in an entirely different world. Now, you might well argue that many of the other aspects of the near-death experience we've discussed, such as drifting out of body or seeing a weird light, could be placed in this category as well. And of course you would be right.

49

But sometimes there's a deeper or at least an additional sense of the supernatural or extradimensional, which includes some of these other factors but goes beyond them. The feeling may not even be tied down to anything that can be readily expressed, but may just put the person in the position of having to say, as many of our interviewees did, "It's hard to put this into words."

In this regard, one strange, otherworldly experience related to us by a doctor of internal medicine who practices in Virginia went like this: "I was in an intensive care unit and not expected to live. I seemed to see, in a hazy, grayish environment, former dead members of my family. Also, there were many apparently injured and crippled people. It was a rather peaceful, tranquil, thought-stimulating, reflective environment.

"I was apparently in that state for several hours, according to medical observers who thought I was dying or would die. I only read about others having similar experiences to this *after* my own event."

Many of the other attempts to describe an otherworldly series of events or impressions were even more nebulous than this. But the next, the eighth, type of positive extradimensional experience we encountered was rather specific in almost all the reports we received. I'm referring to the presence of some sort of special being or beings during the person's extraordinary adventure.

8. A feeling that a special being or beings were present during the near-death encounter. The 8 percent of those in a close brush with death who reported this phenomenon sometimes referred to dead relatives whom they recognized, and other times they identified the being as an angel or Jesus Christ.

We'll go into this subject in much more detail in later chapters, when we discuss angels and possible "celestial companionship" in the afterlife. But here are a couple of representative responses that illustrate the general drift of experiences:

One 76-year-old Iowa woman said, "I was real sick with smallpox and had several operations at the same time. My experience was that my pain was gone and it seemed like God had put his arms around me and given me strength and a desire to live, as my family needed me."

In another, much stranger encounter with some sort of beings, a teacher from Maine said that when under an anesthetic during a serious operation, "I had vivid communication with deceased parents and other deceased members of my family. Unusual topics were discussed. I did not see them, but recognized voices. Long after the incident, I realized that perhaps I did not recognize their life forms in the visions.

"I also had three distinct and separate appearances of 'something' in a Connecticut home—no sight, but sounds, pressure and awareness. Unknown to me, a former resident experienced something similar. She researched and discovered a tragedy of youths. I'm not a highly emotional person—rather staid, I think."

The first of this person's experiences, with the presence of a serious operation, came the closest to the typical near-death encounter that may catapult a person into an extradimensional realm. Also, the impact of the anesthetic may have influenced the vision or dream, but the current lack of scientific research prevents us from arriving at any definite conclusions on this issue.

As for the second set of three incidents, they could well have been triggered by anticipatory fear or anxiety, just as we've seen happen sometimes with muggings or with the mere threat of serious injury that never materializes. Or it could have been a figment of the person's imagination, inspired by popular stories of other haunted houses. Once again, at this stage in our study, we can only present the reports we have, with all their strengths and weaknesses.   51

It won't be until we approach the end of our investigation that we'll be in a position to weigh them all and perhaps come to some tentative conclusions about their cumulative meaning.

9. Perception of a tunnel. Although much has been made of the importance of the vision of a tunnel reported by many with a near-death experience, our surveys have shown this element to be a relatively infrequent sort of perception. With only 3 percent of those who came close to death, or less than 1 million adult Americans, reporting this phenomenon, it plays a rather small role in the total picture presented by the near-death occurrences.

Some of the tunnel reports were positive, and thus should be included with the other possible indicators that point to a relatively pleasant extradimensional realm. Other tunnels, as we'll see in our discussion of hell, are more negative.

As a confirmation of the periodic reports of tunnel experiences, one Pennsylvania psychiatrist told us, "prior to the publication of books in this area, two patients described the tunnel experience to me."

A more immediate, firsthand example of a tunnel experience, which apparently didn't involve a near-death incident but did involve a physical crisis, happened in a dentist's chair. A middle-aged Wisconsin woman related this account: "While in a dentist's chair after having Novocaine, I passed out and seemed to go through a dark tunnel. Then, there was a light, and I saw the Virgin Mary. I don't know exactly what else happened. Could have been a hallucination."

In a more specific, graphic kind of account, an Indiana psychologist said that after a close brush with death through inhaling deadly car fumes, she embarked upon an out-of-body trip and then "saw many lights, which got brighter and brighter at one point—like going down a tunnel."

Some have also reported that the tunnel swirls or seems to be in constant motion. Still others refer in great detail to an opening at the end of the tunnel where a friendly being or perhaps a pleasant, peaceful bucolic scene awaits them.

But from a scientific viewpoint, what, if anything, might these tunnel perceptions mean?

A variety of possible explanations of this phenomenon have been offered. For example, some have suggested that the immediate presence of danger or threat to one's life may conjure up some memory of the security of the mother's womb—hence the movement through a tunnel, back to the ultimate security that existed before birth.

Others have proposed a much more pragmatic explanation: The swirling sensation in some of the tunnel experiences is nothing more than the dizziness that may accompany a half-conscious state. The perception of being in a tunnel, with dark walls bearing in on all sides and from top and bottom, may be nothing more than a preliminary stage just prior to unconsciousness, when the senses such as sight and hearing are shutting down (somewhat like what happens when a television screen loses its picture gradually around the edges as the tube goes out).

But some of the most fascinating suggestions tie the tunnel in to concepts from physics and astronomy, like the black hole in space and the so-called worm hole. Nobody knows quite what the complete significance of these phenomena is, though there has been considerable speculation that one or both of these ripples, warps or "holes" in the universe may in fact be entrances or passageways into a parallel universe that exists alongside our own. If such ideas turn out to be even partially true, the argument goes, it may be that those who encounter a tunnel in their near-death experiences may actually be entering a hole in this universe that may lead to another.

In a related development, there has been considerable

thought among some religious thinkers, such as scientist-theologian Kenneth Boa, that heaven may actually be a multidimensional universe that exists next to our own and occasionally spills over into ours. In other words, we function in a three-dimensional reality and for the most part can understand the universe only in three-dimensional terms (height, width and depth). But there may be another universe—or heaven—that not only encompasses our three dimensions but also many more that we can't even begin to understand.

10. Premonitions of some future event or events. Just as the minds of those in many near-death encounters are expanded or molded to accommodate new dimensions of time or perception, so also there is occasionally a tendency for the person's thought patterns to be jarred out of the present altogether. In those cases, a flash of insight into some future event may be the result.

For example, some of the people in our study reported that during near-death encounters or other related experiences, they learned of events that were in the process of happening at some distance or would happen in the future.

A middle-aged Pennsylvania housewife reported a pattern of strange extradimensional adventures at different points in her life, at least one involving knowledge of events that she could not have known about under ordinary circumstances.

"Twice, in very close calls in automobile accidents, I have had a vivid experience of my life literally rolling backwards before my eyes at a great speed.

"Also, while undergoing a Caesarean section under emergency circumstances and being in very poor physical condition, I had an experience of being in the room with myself, but standing apart from everything going on. I did not care what happened, and felt that it was very unimportant."

54

On a third occasion, which was apparently permeated with anxiety and stress, she said, "I have had the experience of having a member of the family die out of town. I was out of my home for hours while they were trying to contact me. Upon entering my home with no one else at home, the man who had died called out my name clearly and plainly. I thought he was in the house and answered him. After searching the house for him, I became very frightened until the phone call came, saying he was dead."

Premonitions, of course, frequently occur in circumstances other than a close brush with death or a particularly stressful time in the person's life. Some people claim to have extrasensory perception experiences and premonitions on a regular basis, whether they are under stress or not. But still, for a few people, the verge-of-death happening does definitely seem to act as an impetus for making the person's mind perform in highly unusual ways.

These, then, are the ten major positive categories into which our findings can be divided. It would certainly be inaccurate and misleading to equate these groups of experiences directly with heaven because at this stage of research, it's impossible to say with certainty what these adventures we've recounted represent. There are definite similarities to some of the descriptions of heaven we included at the beginning of this chapter.

For example, take the New Testament descriptions of the "resurrection body" in which Jesus made his after-death appearances, and the "heavenly body" and more complete mental understanding and knowledge that the Apostle Paul says believers will have in the afterlife. There are many parallels between these descriptions and the increased mental powers and physical mobility that have been reported by those who have undergone near-death adventures.

But what exactly is the connection between these religious concepts and the verge-of-death reports? Have those involved in close brushes with death merely gone through   55 some sort of strange adventure in their minds, rather than in any sort of objective supernatural reality? Or to put it another way, have their experiences tapped some deep reservoirs of the imagination, which represent more of a reflection of their own beliefs and biases about the afterlife than an independent adventure in another superuniverse that some call heaven?

To explore these questions more fully, let's now take a brief look at what the typical American believes about heaven and see how closely these inner presuppositions parallel what is reported actually to happen in a close brush with death.

5

Heaven as
a State of Mind

OUR MINDS ARE CAPABLE of more amazing feats than
most of us are perhaps aware of. So it may be that
a large number of the accounts of extraterrestrial
and supernatural encounters are mere mental
events. In other words, they may occur solely from
such powerful psychological forces as an overwhelming need to fulfill strong inner desires or wishes; certain forms of temporary or ongoing insanity; serious
physical and emotional traumas and stresses; or even
just a natural inclination to tell tall tales.

But can the reports of positive, heavenlike near-
death experiences, such as those we examined in
the previous chapter, be explained in these terms—
by attributing them solely to the imagination? Or
is it possible that they may be based on actual outside observations or other forms of objective
truth?

In attempting to answer these questions, let's first
turn our attention to what's going on in the minds
of those who have been responding to our near-death
studies. Then, perhaps we'll be in a better position
to speculate about whether or not the reports of

near-death experiences are simply projections of several million vivid imaginations.

We've surveyed a national sample of the American people to ascertain the details of their beliefs and attitudes toward life after death. One consistent, overwhelming belief that pervades our studies and that probably has been a commonly held assumption by most humans since prehistoric times is that heaven does, indeed, exist.

At the Gallup Poll, we've asked national audiences in 1952, 1965 and 1980 this question: "Do you think there is a Heaven, where people who have led good lives are eternally rewarded?"

A consistent seven out of ten people have responded "yes," and there is every reason to believe that the number would have been at least as high in earlier years, when religious faith was more pervasive.

But even though this tendency of Americans to believe in heaven has remained at about 70 percent of the total population for the last 30 years, there are some interesting variations in belief, depending on such factors as the person's education, sex, religion and place of residence.

First of all, more women than men believe in heaven, by 75 percent to 66 percent. This orientation of the female toward faith is a characteristic that permeates our entire study, and it's important to keep this fact in mind, especially if it sometimes seems we are relying heavily on accounts and experiences of women.

Also, there's a big difference in beliefs among those living in different geographical locations. If you live in the Northeast or the Far West and find yourself running into relatively few people who believe in heaven, your experience may be quite typical of your region. We've found that only 61 percent of the people in the East and 58 percent of westerners believe in heaven, while 76 percent of those in the Midwest and an incredible 84 percent of people in the South believe. That figure in the South, by the way, goes up to 89 percent for those who live in the Deep South.

There's also a tendency for beliefs in heaven to increase in direct proportion to how little education a person has. So we've discovered that about six in ten of those with a college education believe, while a much larger 77 percent of those educated only through grade school do.

But even though there is a big difference in beliefs according to educational level, there's no substantial difference between young people and their elders. You might think that the older you get, the more likely you are to begin to think about—and believe in—the pearly gates. But actually, we've found that the highest response for belief in heaven—more than 75 percent—came from young people from 18 to 24 years of age.

Finally, as might be expected, the intensity of belief in heaven increases as personal religious experience increases. An overwhelming 86 percent of those with a deep religious experience say they believe in heaven, while a more modest 64 percent of those without such an experience believe.

But we've also come up with some findings on the religious front that you might not expect—namely, that there's been a steady decline during the last 30 years in Roman Catholics who believe in heaven. When we first asked our question about heaven in 1952, 83 percent of Catholics said they believed, but now that figure is down to 73 percent. Protestants, on the other hand, have shown a steady conviction about heaven, with 75 percent saying they believed back in 1952, and 77 percent saying "yes" in our most recent 1980 survey.

We'll see later on that Roman Catholic belief in other aspects of the afterlife has declined over the years, and at the same time, Protestant convictions have intensified. Part of the reason for the upsurge in Protestant belief may be the growing born-again or evangelical movement. With its stress on biblical authority and traditional Christian doc- 59 trine, this movement has had a significant impact among Protestants during the last couple of decades.

These, then, are the general outlines of the types of people who believe in heaven in this country. Now, let's fill in some of the details to see exactly what they believe.

First of all, where is heaven?

As might be expected, many people say they think of it as "up there," or "in the vast up-above." When pressed to be more specific, though, they tend to place heaven outside this universe. As one 65-year-old Georgia woman told us, "It's so far away. I think we always think of it as 'up,' and I would say it's in the vast up-above somewhere. But I don't think it's physical. And I don't think it's on another planet."

A sophisticated, extra-time approach emerged in some conversations we had. One woman from Arizona, for example, said she thought heaven was "another dimension." And a 39-year-old New York businessman, picking up on this theme, put it this way: "I get the sense it will be a totally different kind of experience from what we have on earth. There will be more dimensions to reality in heaven. Now, our lives are three-dimensional. But then, they may be 20-dimensional. Our consciousnesses will be greatly expanded."

These responses are reminiscent of some of the reports and descriptions we received from those with near-death experiences, and they also bring to mind certain interpretations we offered of those experiences. For example, as we've already mentioned, scientist-theologian Kenneth Boa indicates in his writings that heaven may be an extradimensional realm existing as a kind of parallel universe to our own. In other words, heaven and its inhabitants may exist at times in part of our three-dimensional space, but the total reality of the afterlife would extend far beyond our own.

To illustrate this concept, Boa cites a book called *Flatland*, which was written by Edwin Abbott in the nineteenth century. In this fable, the people of Flatland have only two dimensions, width and depth, but they don't have height. As a result, if a three-dimensional creature such as a human being enters their space, all they can see is that part of the person's body cutting across the flat plane of their reality.

It's somewhat like the experience of the person who puts on goggles and submerges himself exactly to eye level in a still pool of water. If in some way the person could be prevented from seeing below or above the water but was able to see only at eye level, along the surface, he would get an idea of what the Flatlanders are and are not able to see.

In a similar way, a professional designer told us, "I think heaven is within me in a sense. I think it's the spirit world, and you can't compare the spiritual and material dimensions. You don't cross over from one to the other at a definite place because they often merge together. When I get to heaven, I may recognize that I've been there already, that it's been inside me all along."

This kind of speculation about where heaven is can be provocative, but the chances are we'll ultimately always be left with a considerable mystery as long as we're only talking about what people believe, and not what they've actually experienced.

So in the long run, perhaps it's best, when asked in the abstract, "Where is heaven?" not to get too serious. Or, perhaps, to respond as one person did in our survey, "It's not in Brooklyn!" Or as another said, "I have no earthly idea!"

Even if there isn't much agreement or certainty as to where heaven is, people often seem more in accord about when you enter it. Many believe that you enter heaven at death, though sometimes there may be a delay. These 61 individuals suggest that there may be a holding place of some sort, or what we have already called a vestibule on the periphery of heaven, before you get all the way into God's extradimensional realm. A few call this preliminary place paradise, after Jesus' promise to the thief on the cross, "Today shalt thou be with me in Paradise" (Luke 23:43). Others might refer to it as purgatory.

Many of these general beliefs are quite similar to the reports we received from those who had unusual near-death encounters.

What does the average American believe the landscape of heaven may be like? We asked a national cross section of people several questions about the nature of heaven, including how they think the afterlife will differ from their present lives and also whether certain words or terms apply to their beliefs about life after death, or heaven.

Here, with a few representative comments, are the main ways people feel that a positive afterlife experience will be different from this life.

• The afterlife will be a *better life and a good life.*
• There will be *no more problems or troubles.* "No trials and tribulations . . . worries and cares will vanish . . . no worries, no cares, no sorrows. I think to be worried all the time would really be awful."
• There will be *no more sickness or pain.*
• The afterlife will be a *spiritual, not a physical realm.* "Totally spiritual . . . lack of physical limitations . . . there's not going to be a three-dimensional experience."
• It will be *peaceful.* "I think we'll be more peaceful because you really live your hell on earth."
• The afterlife will be *happy and joyful, no sorrow.*

In another part of our survey, when we asked people to pick what they believed to be the most likely characteristics of heaven, more than half affirmed each of these responses.

- Heaven will be peaceful.
- Those who make it to heaven will be happy.
- They will be in the presence of God or Jesus Christ.
- There will be love between people
- God's love will be the center of life after death.

Happiness, peace, love and the presence of God or Christ—those qualities will permeate the atmosphere of heaven. In a sense, just as we breathe in air, the inhabitants of heaven will inhale and exhale love.

But this is only the beginning of the picture the general public paints of heaven. At least a quarter of those surveyed also listed these features of the afterlife.

- Crippled people will be whole.
- People in heaven will grow spiritually.
- They will see friends, relatives, or spouses.
- They will live forever.
- There will be humor.

So now we're beginning to flesh out this picture of heaven that exists in the corporate mind of the American people. You won't see anybody with a disease or physical handicap in heaven—all will be physically perfect. There will also be some camaraderie with old friends and relatives, an eternal continuity of personal relationships from this present life.

A good 25 percent said they believe there will be humor in heaven. They were usually unable or unwilling to explain exactly what they meant by this, but perhaps they had in mind some sort of enjoyable heavenly comedy act, such as that suggested by George Burns in the movie *Oh God!*

The conviction that those in heaven will be able to grow spiritually is held by more than a third of all adult Americans, or about 50 million people.

A substantial number of people believe that the afterlife is a dynamic place or dimension where there's a lot of activ-   63 ity and action. Or as one young Texas woman put it, "I don't believe we'll just be sitting around, playing harps and singing to each other!"

To be more precise, about one in five of those polled responded:

- People in heaven will grow intellectually.
- They will have responsibilities.
- They will minister to the spiritual needs of others.
- Those in heaven will be recognizable as the same people that they were on earth.
- There will be angels in heaven.

So now we have a population of heaven interacting with one another in a constant state of change, growth and service to others. Not only that, in some way these individuals are recognizable as they were on earth, but their relationships with others have now expanded to include celestial companions of some sort.

So this is what heaven would look like if we were looking through the eyes of the "typical" American, but so far, our view is still at a great distance. We know generally what heaven is like, but what about the specifics?

Remember: We're still only talking about personal beliefs, *not* about reports that purport to be actual experiences in close brushes with death and related incidents.

A number of people we talked to saw heaven as a kind of Garden of Eden. One woman from Illinois said, "The picture I get is that it will be a perfect place, where the blind see and crippled people can walk. There will be trees, no pollution, fresh water—some of the characteristics of a Garden of Eden."

Another woman from the Midwest also started out with a rather traditional view of heaven's landscape, but then her descriptions began to get more unusual: "I think it's eternal happiness, being reunited with old friends and relatives and loved ones. I envision people dressed differently

64

than on earth—perhaps in robes. But I don't think there will be trees. In fact, I think heaven will be completely different, not like earth at all. This is thought-provoking. I think it will be bright and sunny, and I suppose I can't help but say fleecy clouds and that sort of thing. I don't think there will be a need for shelter, though, because there won't be any threat from the elements."

Some of the descriptions of heaven we encountered are so specific and familiar it made me feel as though these people had already been there. One young minister's wife from the Southwest said, "I see a river flowing down the middle of it. There are streets of gold, gardens with fruit trees and probably a lot of vegetation. There's also some type of wall with precious stones, and I imagine some type of city. The Bible talks about mansions where we live, and I also see a lot of water—maybe the 'living water' Jesus said He would give us."

An elderly woman from the Deep South seemed to be thinking of heaven as the perfect fulfillment of her own later years here on earth because she said, "Heaven is the place where we go to retire, eternal retirement. I think when God created the earth, He put things down here much like they are there. The difference is that there, there won't be sin. Everything will be perfect, the way He wanted the earth to be to begin with. Perfect trees and animals, with the whole thing similar to the way it is here on earth, except a lot prettier. I think our environment here on earth is a kind of model, but a shadowy, imperfect one, of the way things will be in heaven."

Several other people picked up on this idea of the physical setting of heaven being a perfect, unpolluted environmentalists' dream. One woman from the Midwest focused on the animals she believes will reside in heaven: "I believe when Adam and Eve sinned, all the universe fell, and death came into the world then. Before that, animals and trees and all other living things had eternal life. Nothing died.   65

Then, all of a sudden death came into the world with our disobedience to God. So my theory is that at the time of redemption, when we go to heaven, everything will be restored—lions, dogs, insects. Once again, nothing will die."

But does this mean animals have souls? we asked.

"No," she replied, "because I don't think the animals have a choice, whether they choose to live one way or the other. I mean, it wasn't God's intention for animals to die, just as it wasn't His intention for man to die. So when redemption is complete, I believe maybe the animals will be restored, with no death. God will recreate them as part of a new Garden of Eden. And who knows? Heaven might even be like C. S. Lewis's *Narnia*, where the animals talk!"

Fascinated with the comprehensive mental picture she was painting, we pressed her further: Will the redeemed humans in heaven eat the redeemed animals?

"No!" she said. "Of course, the Bible talks about the feasts in heaven, but humans didn't eat animals in the first Garden of Eden. They were vegetarians. It was after Noah that God gave them permission to eat animals. So I think there will be banquets in heaven that don't require us to kill any animals."

Here's the way one young man from New Jersey summarized the idea of heaven possessing a perfection that our present surroundings only suggest: "All of heaven will have the quality of the most beautiful earthly experiences. There is a sense in which man reflects the image of God, and I would say by the same token earth was in some sense made in the image of heaven. So our beautiful flowers reflect the perfect flowers of heaven. Our best constructed and maintained streets and thoroughfares are a reflection of the 'streets of gold' the Bible talks about in the afterlife."

Although many of these descriptions are earth-oriented, in the sense that they are expressed in language and concepts we associate with our present existence, some people go far beyond our physical experiences in their beliefs.

For example, a 35-year-old woman from New England said, "I don't think heaven will be a place with big pearly gates. Physical surroundings don't interest me—and I think what we see and experience there will be so different from what we know in this life that it's impossible to put it into human words.

"For one thing, I believe we won't be bound by earthly conceptions of time. People are always pressed for time to do things in this life, but it won't be that way in heaven. You'll have more than enough time to do all you want to do or dream of doing. And I think in heaven we'll mainly experience what we think of on earth as a mental existence. I don't think it will be physical, in the sense of my having a mansion so I can live next door to you.

"In some sense, I'll be with you or anybody else I want to be with just by *thinking* about it or *willing* it. And I'm not just talking about some sort of teletransportation, where my body would go from one place to another when I want it to, because I don't think heaven will be primarily a physical experience, as we think of it on the earth. In some sense, I'll have understanding of anything I want to understand, and I'll relate to anyone I want to relate to, just as a part of my natural state of being in heaven."

As she said, it's hard to put some things into human language when there's no language or experience to express what an extradimensional reality may be like. Along these same lines, listen to what one man from Florida had to say about the strange reality of heaven:

"When I think about what we might look like in heaven, I get images that are totally different from anything I know in this life. For example, when an infant dies and goes to be with God, will we encounter that little person as a baby in the afterlife?

"I really don't think so. I think his spirit might blossom into the fullness that he *might* have been if he had only lived on to maturity on earth. Yet, if that were my child   67 that died, I still think I'd recognize him when we meet after death. Maybe it's as though we each have certain facets of our personalities that develop fully at different ages, and when we're still on earth, we can only see traces of personality traits that came before or will come to fruition later.

"But in heaven, we'll see each person as a kind of spiritual prism, with all sorts of surfaces and angles which we can study in their full beauty, all at once. So if my baby dies, I'll still be able to see him as a baby. But I'll also see what he *could* have been on earth, and possibly will become or has become in heaven."

In our survey of basic beliefs, 11 percent said they thought people will be the same age as they were when they died, but this man from Florida doesn't quite fit into this group. In his view, people will in a sense be the same age as they were when they died, but at the same time, they'll be every other age they were or could have been.

These, then, are the major outlines and details of what American adults believe about heaven. Now, how are we to interpret these attitudes in light of the reports by those who have had near-death encounters?

First of all, let's examine how these beliefs compare with actual near-death experiences.

Those who had a brush with death or a related experience sometimes reported an out-of-body experience. Nothing quite like that comes out in the general beliefs about heaven, though there is a pervasive assumption that those in heaven will have some sort of "body" which is recognizable or resembles their body on earth.

People near death were able to see and hear exceptionally well, and the public's beliefs coincide with these experiences. Those close to death sometimes had an overwhelming sense of peace and painlessness, and that's what is generally believed about heaven by those we surveyed.

68 Those on the verge of death also sometimes saw lights

or bright lights, but this was only mentioned occasionally in the in-depth surveys we conducted about beliefs on the afterlife. A quick review of one's life was one of the more common aspects of a near-death experience, but wasn't mentioned at all among the beliefs about heaven.

Those near death occasionally had a strange sensation, as though they were in another world, and this is quite consistent with some of the convictions people hold about the "wholly other," unearthly characteristics of heaven. Our near-death reports also included references to the presence of a being or beings of various types, and beliefs about heaven likewise include a large and varied population.

On the other hand, some of those reporting a near-death incident said they entered or saw some sort of tunnel, but there was no such phenomenon mentioned in the general beliefs survey. (We'll see in a later chapter on hell, however, the tunnel does come up in a more disturbing context.)

Finally, premonitions sometimes accompanied near-death experiences. Although this kind of supermental activity wasn't mentioned specifically among the general beliefs about heaven, there was a solid conviction among many people that their intellectual powers would be increased in heaven and that they would understand much more fully things that they only partially comprehend now.

So what can we conclude when we compare the reports of near-death experiences with the general beliefs of the average person about heaven?

For one thing, the general beliefs are not necessarily inconsistent with the concrete near-death reports. And in some cases what people say they believe about heaven actually coincides with what others say they have experienced.

On the other hand, there are also many areas where the beliefs of the public and the reports of specific verge-of-death experiences *don't* overlap. In other words, people who come close to death or undergo some similar stressful situation frequently have mystical kinds of encounters that   69 go beyond, but don't necessarily conflict with, what the average person says he believes.

In trying to determine whether we should attach any significance or meaning to these similarities and differences, it will be helpful to consider briefly how this whole subject relates to a couple of fascinating topics: 1) arguments purporting to prove the existence of God or heaven; and 2) wish fulfillment, or projection of mental images in such a way that they appear to be real, but actually are not.

Years ago, religious philosophers would have argued that the pervasiveness of beliefs about heaven was some sort of proof there *is* a heaven. Here's a typical way some of those arguments were made.

All human beings have certain longings and needs, and it's reasonable to assume that if we desire something very deeply, the object of that desire must exist someplace. There is ample proof of this principle in the verifiable physical world. Our hunger points to the existence of food; our thirst points to water; our sex drive points to sexual union. By the same token, our spiritual longings, fears and ideas may point to God, heaven and the other aspects of the spiritual realm.

We sense intuitively and often firmly believe that there is some spiritual reality beyond the physical world. At the same time, we long to understand what it's all about and to reach a level of certainty about such ultimate questions as the existence of God. As a result, the argument goes, the very fact that we possess these deep drives and feelings is proof of the existence of their spiritual objects.

This sort of argument doesn't carry as much weight these days as it did among the theologians of the Middle Ages. But even some modern religious thinkers and philosophers hold that our pervasive beliefs about the spiritual dimension can help us understand a little more about God.

For example, the liberal Roman Catholic theologian Hans Kung says at one point in his *Does God Exist?*, "Belief

70

in God is a gift. Reality exists before me. If I do not cut myself off, but open myself entirely to reality as it opens out to me, then I can accept in faith its primary ground, its deepest support, its ultimate goal: God. . . ."

Kung stresses that people have sometimes come to believe there's a God just by His revelation in day-to-day reality and nature. In making this point, he cites one of our 1975 Gallup polls as being "illuminating" in showing the pervasiveness of the sense of a conviction of God's reality. In that survey, 94 percent of Americans said they believed in God.

If you accept this argument that a general belief in God and heaven is at least some evidence of their existence, then some, but not all of the beliefs that have emerged in our surveys may be used to reinforce the validity of *some* of the mystical near-death experiences we've described. The near-death accounts that go beyond or aren't included in the general public beliefs must stand alone—unexplained, but perhaps reflecting a side of the supernatural that we can only know when we come into direct contact with it.

A second possible use of our data is diametrically opposed to this proof-of-God approach. I'm referring to the interpretation that the near-death experiences are a wish fulfillment or projection of concepts and mental pictures that exist solely in people's minds. In other words, the beliefs in our general surveys have been projected in some way into the minds of those who think (erroneously) that they have experienced something special in a close brush with death.

In the last analysis, however, neither of these positions gives us a solid, definitive explanation. The most we can say about the general beliefs on heaven is that they offer some interesting comparisons with the near-death accounts. But to understand more about what happens during a close brush with death, it's necessary to turn back once more to an examination of the close calls themselves.

6

Descent into
the Abyss

THE TERM "afterlife" is often used synonymously
with "heaven" or "paradise" to denote some sort
of pleasant, enjoyable, exciting extradimensional
realm. In other words, when a person dies, he or
she moves automatically into some sort of union with
God or Ultimate Reality or Ground of Being. Any
other state of continuing existence is unthinkable
for many people.

But just as there is good and evil on earth, so
the nagging suspicion persists that some aspects of
the afterlife, for whatever reason, may not be so
nice. To put it in the crassest terms, what about the
abyss, the inferno, the eternal death or estrangement
from God—what about hell?

As might be expected, hell is not a very popular concept among the general public. One indication of this fact is that a significantly smaller number of people, both in this country and abroad,
say they believe in hell than in heaven. In 1952,
1965 and 1981, we asked a national sampling of
American adults this same question: "Do you think
there is a Hell, to which people who have led

bad lives and die without being sorry are eternally damned?"

The results were quite consistent: In 1952, 58 percent replied "yes," they believed in hell. In 1965, 54 percent said "yes." And in 1980, 53 percent replied in the affirmative. These figures are considerably lower than the consistent seven out of ten who said they believed in heaven in those years.

Another interesting fact that emerged from our special survey for this book concerns the backgrounds of those who do or don't believe in hell. Those from the South tend to have the strongest beliefs in hell, with 72 percent saying "yes," they definitely believe. This figure goes up even higher in the Deep South, with 81 percent responding in the affirmative. In the West, on the other hand, belief in hell dips to 36 percent of the population; and in the East, with 41 percent as believers, convictions about the existence of hell aren't much higher.

As is the case with beliefs in heaven, the higher the educational level of the person, the less likely he is to believe in hell. The proportions of those believing in hell climb from 47 percent for those with a college education to 63 percent for those with only a grade school background. Also, significantly more Protestants (61 percent) believe in hell than Catholics (48 percent).

The disbelief in hell gets even more dramatic when you examine attitudes in other countries. In 1968, for example, we asked people in this country and also in eight foreign countries the simple question, "Do you believe in hell?"

The positive response in the United States, at 65 percent, was higher than in other years, probably because the question was posed with fewer qualifications than in other surveys. But the level of belief in most other countries, with Greece being the only exception, was considerably lower than in the U.S. Here is a summary of our findings:

Question: "Do you believe in hell?"

	YES	NO	NO OPINION
	%	%	%
United States	65	29	6
Greece	62	25	13
Norway	36	45	19
Finland	29	49	22
Netherlands	28	61	11
Austria	26	68	6
Switzerland	25	67	8
West Germany	25	62	13
Great Britain	23	58	19
France	22	70	8
Sweden	17	71	12

This tendency of a large proportion of the public in many foreign nations not to believe in hell stands in stark contrast to the traditional teachings of Christianity, which is the major organized religion in these countries. The New Testament, of course, takes the clear position that there *is* a hell where, as Jesus puts it, "men will weep and gnash their teeth" (Matthew 8:12, RSV).

There have been numerous reasons offered as to why so many more people believe in heaven than in hell. One rather provocative response we've heard is, "Hell is like death—people try not to think about it." There are also popular arguments against hell that go like this: "I believe that God is basically good and loving, and I can't imagine such a deity would send anybody off to eternal punishment."

Whatever the arguments, pro and con, many among the general public in the so-called Christian nations have elected to depart from traditional scriptural doctrines. Interestingly enough, this tendency to downplay hell is reflected even more dramatically in our surveys of those who report near-death experiences.

First of all, even though 53 percent of the general population in the United States believe in hell, only about 47 percent of those with near-death experiences believe. This disparity might indicate that the verge-of-death encounter was, for most people, sufficiently positive that they felt they had less reason to fear negative consequences in the after-life.

In support of this thesis, our major national poll of those who had a close brush with death showed that only one percent said that they "had a sense of hell or torment." Similarly sparse references to hell-like experiences in other near-death studies have led some researchers to conclude that hell must not play much of a role in the afterlife. But a closer examination of our own surveys and interviews makes us believe that the picture is more complex than that.

For example, in the major survey we did on those with near-death experiences, 15 percent of all adult Americans, or about 23 million people, said they had had a close brush with death. But only slightly more than 30 percent of those people related anything positive about their experiences. The others either just described the horror and pain of their accident or illness, or had something else negative to say.

Also, in a follow-up survey, which included many in-depth questions about these experiences, we asked every-one, "Do you feel that you actually had a glimpse of an afterlife or Heaven, or not?"

A total of 18 percent responded "yes, definitely," that they had glimpsed heaven or the afterlife; and another 11 percent said, "yes, maybe" they had—for a total positive response of 29 percent. But a solid 28 percent gave a definite "no," they hadn't glimpsed heaven or the afterlife; 17 per-cent said they couldn't say; and the final 26 percent gave no response. In other words, even among those who re-ported a close brush with death, less than a third saw the experience as even *possibly* related to heaven; and only 18 percent seemed certain they had been in contact with a heavenly realm.

There was a similar breakdown when those with a near-death encounter were asked, "Did you feel that you were in the presence of God or Jesus Christ, or not?" A total of 21 percent said "yes, definitely"; 8 percent said "yes, maybe"; 25 percent said "no"; 15 percent said they couldn't say; and 31 percent gave no response.

There are several possible inferences we can draw from these responses. First of all, people are quite careful about making the claim that they've had a direct encounter with heaven or with God. In fact, one of the elements that stood out in our studies was the precision of the responses. Very few of the answers smacked of a rote, doctrinaire kind of attitude. Most people tried to describe exactly what had happened to them, and they seemed to want to let the reader draw his or her own conclusions from the facts that were presented. In other words, they weren't particularly interested in grinding any favorite axes.

But what about the fact that such a relatively large number indicated that they either hadn't experienced heaven or couldn't say one way or the other?

Of course, it wouldn't be appropriate to conclude automatically that just because a person didn't sense the presence of God or heaven, he must therefore have been involved with hell. But it does seem clear that many of these people had either a neutral or negative experience that caused them to exclude the presence of God or some heavenly dimension in their evaluations of the incident. At any rate, they were reluctant to interpret their experience in positive terms.

To understand this point better, let's look more closely at several near-death experiences that contain some negative elements and attempt to determine what they may mean for our study.

In one report we received, a 30-year-old Maryland investor said, "I had an operation—four-and-a-half hours. I was under, and I felt I was dying. I felt I was being tricked into death. In my mind, I was fighting with faces unknown to me, and I felt I had to have all my wits about me, to keep from dying. I continued to fight for some time. But as in a dream, which can seem hours, it might have been only seconds.

"I remember not breathing, and strange colors, lights and designs took shape in my brain. Later, I felt relieved and woke up in the recovery room. I had stopped breathing on the operating table and was revived, I was told. I knew I had stopped breathing, and I knew I was near death, even though I had been under."

This experience was clearly quite negative, and the man who was involved explicitly recognized this fact. When asked if he felt he had had a glimpse of heaven or of God, he responded with a resounding "no!"

His perceptions while he was going through his close brush with death are susceptible to a number of possible interpretations. First of all, one might immediately say that the unknown faces around him were merely vague perceptions of the medical personnel surrounding him during the operation. Similarly, the strange colors and designs might have been due to the lack of oxygen getting to his brain when he stopped breathing.

The problem with this explanation is that it presupposes a fuzzy, semiconscious state, yet this man recalls being quite lucid as he battled with whoever or whatever was trying to trick him into death. With great clarity and concentration, he fought and used his wits to keep from dying.

A more likely interpretation would seem to be that he found himself on the verge of extinction; there was some sort of volitional and personal quality in the evil that he was facing; and he realized instinctively that he had to marshal all his inner resources to fight back, to keep from going over the edge.

There's a certain primeval quality about this perception of death as a seductive adversary—and the need to battle against it at all costs to survive. Since the earliest times, for example, people in cold climates have been warned that if they find themselves getting sleepy while out trudging through a snowstorm, it's important to fight ferociously against feelings of relaxation, well-being and sleepiness—because those can be the first signs of freezing and death.

The Apostle Paul made no bones about his own position when he wrote, "The last enemy to be destroyed is death" (1 Cor. 15:26, RSV). And the biblical prince of death and destruction, Satan, is described elsewhere in the Scriptures as "the deceiver of the whole world"—an interesting tie-in with our Maryland investor's feeling that he was being tricked.

Let's turn next to a middle-aged Illinois housewife who was very ill with double pneumonia: "My fever was 104 degrees—this was about seven years ago, and here in my own home. I slept most of the time for about the first three days with the fever. The only time I was awake was when my husband would bother me and change sheets on my bed.

"Other than that, I would [see] huge things coming toward me, like animals with baseball bats. Then, I'd be in this blue-green water, and out in front of me was this huge white, marblelike rock. At the top of the rock was this bright light, and as I got closer to the rock, I saw an image of a person standing on top of it in white clothing—like a robe. But I couldn't tell if it was male or female—I couldn't see the face at all."

This woman said she couldn't say whether this experience involved heaven or God. And from the sound of it, with the huge animals with baseball bats running toward her, it appears to have been anything but enjoyable or pleasant. The bright light and figure on the rock are relatively neutral, neither good nor bad. But the faceless quality of the robed being she encountered seems typical of some negative near-death experiences.

In a similar vein, a young prelaw student in his early twenties reported, "We were on our way to North Dakota for Christmas. My fiancée was in the car, and her sister was driving. We hit some ice and went over a 230-foot embankment. My fiancée and I were thrown from the car, and she miraculously only suffered a broken rib. Her sister was killed.

"As for me, I had been sleeping on the passenger side of the car in the front seat when the car began to skid. My fiancée's sister screamed, but I was never really completely awake. I was aroused, startled, and my main reaction, as I recall it, was just a relaxed feeling. I sat back and didn't even get tense or put my hands up. I took the collision without trying to protect myself.

"Evidently, I took a good crack on my head because I wasn't myself for about forty-eight hours. During that time, I remember coming to and walking around in the canyon where we had landed. But I couldn't remember getting engaged the night before. I do recall looking up toward the road, about 200 feet above us, where I saw a lot of blinking lights.

"My first thought was, 'I must be dead. This is what death must be.' But it certainly wasn't blissful. Just nothingness. I felt like a piece of protoplasm floating out on the sea. I thought, 'Maybe I'm lost, maybe I'm not going to heaven.'"

Later, after this student was taken to the hospital, he said, "Everything was shadowed over—figures seemed to be moving around me, but I couldn't see facial expressions, only forms. It was so weird. I still thought I must be dead."

Another rather negative report after a near-death incident involved a middle-aged Ohio woman, who said she "collapsed with an asthma attack. I was out six hours and something (would have to be God) said, 'You're dying!' When I came to, I could understand why people were so scared."

In this case, the woman believed that the supernatural presence that communicated to her was God, but the message wasn't all that comforting. Being told she was on the verge of death obviously didn't reassure her at all, and fear rather than joy was the primary emotion that gripped her.

An experience of a kind of void accompanied by mildly unpleasant physical sensations was the main sensation that enveloped one elderly Illinois man after a serious accident: "I died for three minutes. It began with the end of my tongue. I quit breathing. The last thing I remember was numbness in my throat. There was no suffering or ill feeling. But nothing existed, that's all."

It would be hard to argue that this sort of experience is a hell in the conventional sense of the term because there is no gnashing of teeth or searing flames. But at the same time, there is no suggestion that this man's encounter had anything to do with heaven. He seems to have entered a neutral kind of near-death region which was slightly more negative than positive. So if this *was* some sort of supernatural realm, it may be that what he had a taste of was a *vestibule* that stood at the entrance to a more intensely negative dimension of reality.

This mildly negative kind of report is also echoed in other near-death accounts we received.

A 35-year-old Ohio man with an appendix problem told us, "I had gangrene and peritonitis. The poison may have been affecting my mind. I awoke seeing a presence in robes. It had no face. It was not threatening. Much like what one hears of in guardian angels. I even tried to look away, but it stayed.

"The day after this occurrence, the figure appeared again. By this time, I was heavily sedated for pain. This time, it was only there for a few seconds. After my surgery nine days later, I was being wheeled to X-ray after I had a relapse (the bowel kinked off where appendix was re-   81 moved). I felt every small bump and crack as the cart was wheeled along.

"I felt like I was in a great black vacuum. All I could see was my arms hanging onto a set of parallel bars. I knew if I relaxed, my grip on life would cease. It was a complete sense of knowing that life had to be clung to. I knew without any question if I let go, I would die. The feeling of agony of hanging on only lasted a brief while."

This man, a Methodist, told us that "maybe" he had a glimpse of heaven or the afterlife in this experience, but that he definitely didn't feel he was in the presence of God or Jesus Christ. His experience seems, on balance, to be more bad than good because even the nonthreatening faceless being, which he thought might be a guardian angel, was, at best, a neutral presence. This being offered him no clear-cut aid as he was trying to cling to life by what the man perceived as some sort of parallel bars. The man had to use his own power to hang onto his life. As you can see, the behavior of this being was quite different from the comforting beings other people have encountered who offered advice and encouragement.

In some cases, the negative near-death experience also includes a strong feeling of fear. For example, a young supermarket cashier from Mississippi tells this story:

"I was at work, and I got upset and began to cry—until I just stopped breathing. I really could not get any air. I felt I was dying off. I passed out—and I know the Lord was warning me. It was something He was showing me. But it just was not my time to go.

"They rushed me to the hospital. I don't remember going there. But I felt I came to close to dying. For a moment, everyone around me thought I had died. Death was only a step away, but the Lord brought me out of the Darkness. And I thank Him for that because if it was not for the Lord, I would still be out of breath. When I stopped breathing, in my mind the only thing I knew was, 'Lord please save me!' I really felt death."

82

Sometimes, instead of this sense of raw fear, there may be confusion or puzzlement. An elderly California accountant gave this third-person account: "I had an experience with my mother. For several days before her death, she was in a comatose state—no movement of the eyes, no reflexes if touched about the eyes. Yet, when she died, an expression came upon her face that I could read so well. It was as if she were saying, 'What is this that is happening to me?' It was a look of unmistakable puzzlement. There was indeed something happening that was reflected in her facial expression."

This man said that he doesn't believe that this experience gave him a glimpse of heaven, and he didn't sense he was in the presence of God or Jesus Christ. Yet his mother obviously saw something. What might it have been?

Many scientists are quite certain that all this woman and the others are seeing is hallucinations or otherwise physically explainable events during these close brushes with death. We'll go into some of their views in great detail in a later chapter.

To summarize, the negative near-death experiences in our study include some of the following features:

• featureless, sometimes forbidding faces;
• beings who are often merely present, but aren't at all comforting;
• a sense of discomfort—especially emotional or mental unrest;
• feelings of confusion about the experience;
• a sense of being tricked or duped into ultimate destruction; and
• fear about what the finality of death may involve.

We know that the large majority of near-death experiences have been described in neutral or negative terms, but does this necessarily mean they involved hell?

83

Certainly, most of our responses—and that includes

more than six in ten people in our survey who reported coming close to death—merely described their accident or serious illness, without injecting mystical elements into the account. Also, the negative descriptions and evaluations of the near-death experiences were often only mildly negative; or in some cases, they mixed negative and positive elements together.

This scenario may not be quite in line with some pictures of hell as a place of total, unmitigated torment. But at the same time, it's not necessarily inconsistent with many religious concepts of hell.

For example, the New Testament pictures Satan, his followers and all unbelievers as being thrown ultimately into a lake of fire and brimstone (see Rev. 20:7–15) at the end of the age, or human history. But the Bible is rather vague about what happens between the time of death and this final judgment.

The Apostle Paul sometimes refers to followers of Christ as having "fallen asleep" until the last judgment; others have described the state between death and final judgment as a "dreamless sleep." In this condition, the dead awaiting the end of history may be regarded as, in effect, unconscious or unaware of the nature of the afterlife until their ultimate resurrection. On the other hand, in support of immediate transport to heaven (or hell), many people cite such passages as the thief on the cross, who was told by Christ, "Truly, I say to you, today you will be with me in Paradise." (Luke 23:43)

What it comes down to is that Christian theologians and Bible scholars can't agree about what happens to a person immediately after he dies. And that's part of what makes the increasing number of near-death reports so tantalizing. It's quite possible that close brushes with death may briefly open a window on the negative as well as the positive poles of the afterlife. If this is so, then perhaps what we've been glimpsing, in these accounts of unpleasant near-death expe-

84

riences, is something of what the negative side of immortality may be like.

In support of this interpretation, it's helpful to compare our findings with what some leading religious thinkers and philosophers have surmised about the negative, hellish dimension of the afterlife just after death. C. S. Lewis, for example, in his *The Great Divorce,* pictures hell as an empty city, which at first glance seems vaguely depressing and boring, but not necessarily a center of terrible tortures.

But the emotionally devastating aspect of the place gradually comes to light when it becomes clear that the inhabitants—or former inhabitants—of the city just can't get along with each other without quarrelling. As one of Lewis's characters says, "As soon as anyone arrives he settles in some street. Before the week is over he's quarrelled so badly that he decides to move." So the town keeps expanding as people move away from other people, leaving empty houses behind.

Another character explains the antisocial, shrivelled-up nature of hell in these terms: "All Hell is smaller than one pebble of your earthly world: but it is smaller than one atom of *this* world, the Real World [heaven]. Look at yon butterfly. If it swallowed all Hell, Hell would not be big enough to do it any harm or to have any taste. . . . For a damned soul is nearly nothing: it is shrunk, shut up in itself. Good beats upon the damned incessantly as sound waves beat on the ears of the deaf, but they cannot receive it. Their fists are clenched, their teeth are clenched, their eyes fast shut. First they will not, in the end they cannot, open their hands for gifts, or their mouths for food, or their eyes to see."

In other words, the true nature of hell slips up on those unfortunate enough to enter it permanently. It may seem only neutral or mildly negative at first, but it gets worse and worse before you even know what's happening. In the Christian view, the distinctive thing about hell is that it's

85

a state of separation from God—and that is ultimately what Lewis is getting at in his description.

In our general survey of the American public's convictions about the afterlife, those who believe in hell also offered some interesting commentary on what eternal separation from God might be like.

One Arizona woman said she believes that those going to hell will, immediately after death, enter "a tunnel full of roots, full of devils and mean people." And in some parallel accounts related by those who had negative near-death experiences, we also came across a few references to tunnels or caves. In other words, the tunnel concept, which has so often been mentioned in connection with the heavenlike near-death experience, may have a negative as well as a positive application.

Another description of the eternal abyss, which comes quite close to the accounts related by those with near-death experiences, was offered by a New York businessman: "I think it's the opposite of heaven. I think it will be dark, not a sense of light as in heaven. Also, there will be a constant negative deterioration of the personalities of those who go there. Growth is a part of God and heaven, while destruction characterizes hell.

"Also, I don't think there's going to be a lot of camaraderie there. Some people say, 'I don't mind going to hell because there will be a lot of good company there.' But I don't think that's true. I think those in hell will be totally alone. There won't be a lake of fire with many people around—each individual will be by himself. And those in hell will be forced to look within themselves and constantly deal with their most difficult emotions and feelings of hopelessness."

The negative descriptions we received from some of those who came close to death are not as horrendous as the "eternal fire" and similar characteristics of hell to which

86 Jesus and others in the New Testament refer (e.g., Matthew

18:8). But at the same time, our reports picture a kind of unpleasantness that no one in his right mind would choose to experience for any period of time. And if C. S. Lewis, Charles Williams and others who have speculated creatively about the afterlife are correct in assuming that the terrors of an existence without God gradually intensify after death, then perhaps in some of these near-death accounts we are indeed witnessing the first stages of some sort of negative superdimensional reality after death.

But both in religious tradition and also in our near-death reports, the afterlife is comprised of more than just pleasant or unpleasant places, locations or dimensions of reality. We've also seen some indications that each place has a special population that gives it a distinctive character.

7

The Population
of the Afterlife

THE SPECIAL CHARACTER of any place on earth arises from the nature of its people—and the same principle seems to apply to the extradimensional, unearthly adventures reported by those who have apparently had a glimpse of eternity. If the accounts that have been related to us really do reflect some intimations of immortality, they disclose an incredibly rich variety of beings and presences in the afterlife.

When you hear that someone has had an encounter with some sort of eternal, extradimensional reality, one of the first questions that usually comes to mind is, "Who—or what—is in *control* of that reality?"

In a number of the reports we've received, there is a powerful presence, a dominant being or a group of beings who seem to be in charge, directing or advising the person to do or understand certain things. In a number of cases, those who have been close to death describe these beings in traditional religious terms, possibly because this is the only hu-

89

man terminology they have at their disposal to communicate what is essentially an ineffable experience.

To understand the language they are using and be in a better position to sort through that language and come closer to the core of these strange encounters, let's take a brief look at the categories various theologies have used to identify the "lords of life after death."

The afterlife in almost every religion has been populated by fantastic supernatural beings. Islam, as we've already seen, has the one god, Allah, but he is surrounded by an extensive entourage of helpers, such as angels and jinn, or genii, who are a step below angels in power and authority.

Some of these superhuman entities are hardly distinguishable from human beings in appearance, as was the case with the gods of the Greeks, who posed as men and intervened regularly in their affairs. Similarly, the two angels who visited Lot in Sodom and warned him to leave with his family before the city was destroyed are described in terms that make them appear almost as much human as divine.

Others, though, like the Old Testament cherubim and seraphim, are strange and even fearsome creatures. The cherubim, for example, were reported by the prophet Ezekiel to have four faces, four wings and spinning wheels attached to their bodies. Their functions included standing guard over the route to the tree of life in the Garden of Eden, and also supporting God's throne.

The people we interviewed who were involved in near-death encounters or related incidents also reported seeing and interacting with strange beings. Some of these beings were perceived as on a level of God; some on a secondary level of divine assistants (or what some might traditionally call angels) and some on the level of demons or devils. Let's now turn to some specific accounts to see exactly what these individuals actually experienced. Then we'll examine how their reports might be interpreted in light of both ancient and modern knowledge and beliefs about supernatural beings.

One of the most extensive accounts we received came from a nurse who lives in Pennsylvania. Here's the way she described her near-death encounter:

"My experience happened when I was 17 years old, about a week after my daughter's birth. She was born at home, and the doctor ran into problems. He finally had to use forceps and take the baby. I was very ill afterwards, so they sent me to the hospital.

"I was there three days and they wanted to operate. My husband was against this, so he took me home—although I was so ill that I was not able to sit up in bed. It was a Sunday afternoon. He took a taxi and had to carry me in his arms like a baby.

"By the time I got home, it seemed that I got strength—where from, I do not know. But I got out of the cab and walked into the house, up to our third-floor apartment. I changed the bed the way I wanted it. I then undressed and got into bed. I felt wonderful. I had never had a feeling like that before, and never since.

"My family and neighbors were all there because they were dumbfounded to see the miraculous change that had come over me. Then, just as though there was someone talking to me, a voice told me that I was going to die and that I should let my husband and family know.

"So I called them all together in the room. I held my husband's hand and said to them, 'You must all prepare to meet your God because I am now going to meet mine.'

"I felt so peaceful, I didn't have a pain. And when I left the hospital only about three hours before, I was racked with pain. It seemed that I went off in a trance of some kind. While I was in this state, I had a vision.

"It seemed that all these angels came from heaven and, holding hands, they formed a stairway reaching all the way up to heaven. It seemed that as I ascended these stairs   91 up to heaven, I knew everything that was going on in my home. My family and neighbors were crying and my husband was kneeling at the bed, begging God to please spare me for the baby's sake.

"I kept going up this stair of angels' hands until I reached heaven. When I reached the top, there was a great mist before the door, and an angel said to me, 'That mist is your family's prayers for your return. Why don't you ask the Lord to let you come back to raise your child?'

"When I went through the mist, I could see this person sitting on a throne, surrounded by this mist. I said, 'Lord, please let me go back and raise my child.' He did not reply but took my hand and turned me around and led me back to the stairs to descend. In the meantime, I was out so long that the family was making plans for the undertaker and sending telegrams. When I came to, shouting and singing, I am sure you can imagine what kind of a day that was. Well, I was 17 years old. I am 70 now, and I only had the one child, but I have five grandchildren, all grown, and now three great-grandchildren."

This incredibly detailed story should go down as something of a classic in accounts of this type. The only thing that may set it apart from many other near-death accounts is that the woman apparently had an unaccountable relapse after being well on the road to recovery. But it's clear from the reaction of her family when she "returned"—as well as from their crying and grieving while she was unconscious (or temporarily dead)—that they felt they had lost her permanently.

Some of the key extradimensional beings in this incident are graphically portrayed. First of all, there was the bodyless voice that gave her the message she was about to die. Then, there were the hosts of apparently anthropomorphic angels who held hands to form a stairway for her up to heaven. Next, some sort of head angel, who was acting as spokesman for the others, explained to her some of the things that were going on and gave her some advice. Finally, there was a God-like being, whom the woman called Lord, who made the decision to send her back to the world of the living.

This dominant "Lord" figure appears as a prominent personage in a number of other near-death reports. One woman, a grade-school graduate, told us that she came near death when she had a sudden "pleurisy" attack and as a result wasn't able to catch her breath. "I lay down. I didn't [recognize] anyone. While I was out, I saw the Lord, and I talked with him. He was the most beautiful man. He looked like the sun. He came to my bed and was talking to me."

The "Lord" in this report obviously has human physical features in some sense, in that he looked like "the most beautiful man." Also, he was able to communicate with her as any ordinary person would. But at the same time, there was an unearthly quality, a glow or brightness that the woman could only describe by saying, "He looked like the sun."

Generally speaking, some of the beings that people encounter have a sort of helping, nurturing, guiding or warning function. Other beings are in the position of decision-makers, or actually seem to exercise a certain benevolent but absolute power over the destiny of the person.

For example, one woman who was on the verge of death was beset by a great fear that she would be leaving her family at loose ends, in a state of total confusion, if she died. But then she sensed the presence of some supernatural force: "A spiritual being appeared and told me not to fear—that my family would be all right. My understanding of this being's omniscience was very clear."

In this case, the woman's anxieties immediately disappeared, and she felt as though she were in the most secure set of hands imaginable. There was no doubt in her mind that this presence was in control of her destiny and that everything would be all right. And sure enough, she recovered and was able to assume her family duties with as much vigor as she had possessed before her illness.

In another situation, where a Texas man was, by his own report, "close to death," he was ushered into a strikingly beautiful palace. He said, "I heard a voice tell me to spread the word about how beautiful that place was. It was a beautiful place. The man said, 'It is the house of David.' "

Here, the near-death incident was used by the extradimensional being to direct the person to take certain action—to "spread the word"—when he returned to earth and to good health. Once again, the human being was placed under marching orders by some superior presence, but there is no evidence of rebellion or resentment on the part of the human. Rather, he implicitly accepted the leadership role of the superbeing and was more than willing to comply with his instructions.

But even though these supernatural beings may turn up during a near-death encounter, their appearances are not limited to these situations. They may also show themselves during other highly stressful crises.

In one account that was given to us, a strange presence appeared to a grandmother who was sleeping near her grandchild. This woman often spent hours at night in prayer, and so she was quite sensitive to the spiritual realm.

As she was sleeping that night, she was aroused suddenly by something, and when she looked up, she saw this strange creature, "bound up in light but with a human form." The being, which she identified as an angel, said nothing, but pointed urgently toward the room where the woman's grandchild was sleeping in a crib. "I sensed I had to get up immediately and go into my grandson's room," she recalled.

When she did look into the baby's crib, she confronted a horrifying sight: "The baby had been given a glass bottle during the night but had cracked it, and a blade of glass, like a knife, was resting precariously against the child's throat."

This woman believed fervently that her grandchild's life was saved "by an angelic intervention. If he had moved, that would have been it. I think it was his guardian angel that warned me."

But words of guidance of this type don't always have such positive results. Others have reported messages that aren't tied to a clearly discernible supernatural being, but come from a nebulous "something" that tells about some tragedy that later occurs.

One scientist said unequivocally that he doesn't believe in life after death and is convinced that "heaven or hell are right here during the life I live." But he reported, "When I was ten years old, I would wake up at night crying because something told me my mother would die when I became 18. She died, the week after my eighteenth birthday."

The words of this strange presence which brought a message of death are not too far removed from a personalized compulsion toward suicide that gripped another young man during an extremely stressful period of his life.

In this case, the young man, a college student, said, "I was under a compulsion, under such stress that I wanted to commit suicide. I had been attending a series of religious meetings, and one night I had a terrible dream. I woke up with a start, crying out 'Jesus!' and I had a sense this was going to be my day, that something dramatic was going to happen to me.

"I was a little frightened and I spoke to one of the counselors at the conference. He said, 'There's nothing to be afraid of. Jesus is Lord.'

"That day, one of the other people at the conference prayed over me, and they went through some steps in what is known as a 'deliverance.' At that moment, I physically felt something leave my body. It felt like a great weight   95 was being lifted from my chest, and it seemed to come right out of my mouth. From that day on, I never again had a problem with thoughts of committing suicide."

An even more clear-cut encounter with a clearly identifiable, personal force of evil happened to a young Texan who was spending a summer doing volunteer work on an Indian reservation in New Mexico. His story went like this:

"There were only three 'Anglos' there on the reservation, me and my partner John and an older missionary worker. We went to a dance one night, a rain dance, at about two or three in the morning. I didn't realize at first we weren't supposed to be there, but it soon became clear we were off limits when the Indians began to give us strange looks.

"Suddenly for some strange reason, I began to get worried that I might be found dead one morning, so I watched a little longer and then went back to my sleeping quarters. Nothing much happened the next day, but the next night, when my partner and I were asleep in the same room, I woke up. I felt someone standing next to my bed, but I didn't see anything and I became extremely frightened. I tried to scream and wake John up, but I couldn't. I kept sensing this 'being' was saying something to me, but I couldn't understand the message. Even now, though, I distinctly remember saying, 'All right, I promise, I promise!'

"Then, the being left, and the fear was gone, and I could talk again. So I went on back to sleep. But the next day, I was worried about what had happened so I started to pray. I told the Lord what had happened and I said, 'If I've made any promise I shouldn't have, please help me out.'

"But I felt an assurance that there was no difficulty, so I fell off to sleep that night with a sense of confidence. But then I woke up again in the middle of the night—and I felt a hand sliding down my pillow toward my throat. I just said, 'Lord, you take care of it!' and I rolled over and went back to sleep."

This young man never had an experience like this again, but he was convinced he had run into a real demon of some sort. He stressed, though, that he never saw anything during either of these incidents—only sensed the presence of a demonlike creature.

In our surveys, a substantial number of people on every educational level believe that the afterlife will be populated by a hierarchy of clearly identifiable supernatural beings. Other studies we've done can help us refine these figures and beliefs even further. For example, one American in nine (or 11 percent of the general population) believes in ghosts. And despite the larger number of believers in the United States than in other countries on most spiritual issues, as many as 20 percent of the British believe in ghosts, with seven percent reporting they have actually *seen* a ghost!

There also tends to be a distinction in most people's minds between believing in "devils" and *"the* devil." In the most recent poll we've done on this topic, 34 percent of the general adult American public said they believe in the devil as "a personal BEING who directs evil forces and influences people to do wrong." Another 36 percent said they believe in the devil as "an impersonal FORCE that influences people to do wrong." Finally, 20 percent said they didn't believe in the devil at all; and another 10 percent said they were undecided.

In other words, even though a full seven in ten believe in a personal or impersonal devil, only four in ten believe in a host or entourage of devils or demons. It may be that the word "devils" in the plural carries with it the connotation of personal beings that attempt to influence a person's life, or his afterlife, for the worse.

It's also helpful to compare some of the American views on the devil with what people from foreign countries believe because it's altogether too easy for us in the United States to generalize in global terms about our beliefs, 97 when there may be no justification for such generalizations.

Several years ago, we asked the American public the simple question, "Do you believe in the devil?" and in that survey the response was 60 percent "yes," 35 percent "no," and 5 percent "no opinion." Here's how some other nations reacted to the same query:

	YES	NO	NO OPINION
	%	%	%
Greece	67	21	12
United States	60	35	5
Norway	38	44	18
Netherlands	29	57	14
Finland	26	57	17
Switzerland	25	69	6
West Germany	25	62	13
Austria	23	71	6
Great Britain	21	60	19
Sweden	21	68	11
France	17	76	7

As these figures show, after Greece and the United States, belief in a devil drops precipitously in many of the European nations. Why should we have so much more belief in the devil (as well as in heaven, hell, and many other aspects of the afterlife) than do those in these other countries?

For one thing, as we've already indicated in another context, personal faith and religious commitment have been alive and well in America since the founding of the original colonies. Revivals upon revivals have bolstered our beliefs when, at regular intervals, they start to sag.

In recent times, another extremely important factor has been the vitality of a number of grass-roots spiritual renewal movements. These include the charismatic (or neopentecostal) movement, which stresses such spiritual gifts (or *charismata*, to use the New Testament Greek) as speaking in tongues, miraculous healings and prophecies. Other religious forces at work in this country are the evangelical movement and the various born-again movements. Our polls have shown that as many as 50 million adult Americans consider themselves to have had a born-again religious conversion or renewal experience.

All of these overlap, to one extent or another, from movement to movement and religious denomination to denomination, and they have all been responsible for increasing American religious sensitivities significantly during the past two decades. One of the main features of the most powerful and far-reaching Christian spiritual revival movements in the United States, as well as in many foreign countries, has been a stress on the authority of the Bible, including what amounts to a literal acceptance of everything in the Bible as accurate reportage and history.

The implications for these trends are particularly important as we attempt to interpret the various supernatural beings in our near-death and related accounts, because many of the terms and concepts we encounter in people's descriptions are quite consistent with what the Bible portrays. To understand more clearly how the near-death descriptions relate to more formal religious views, let's take a few moments to explore exactly what theology tells us that angels are.

In both the Old and New Testaments, as well as in much of the religious literature outside the Judeo-Christian tradition, angels are considered messengers and special agents of God. For example, an angel told Abraham not to sacrifice his son, Isaac; angels accompanied the Israelites through the wilderness after they left Egypt; and they "were ascending and descending" the ladder that Jacob dreamed about as he received a special message from God about his great future and that of his descendants.

In this regard, it's interesting that in every case we've encountered, those who told us they've had dealings with   99 angels say these beings acted as guides, messengers or protectors. The case of the Pennsylvania nurse who says she ascended to heaven on a ladder formed by angels is particularly instructive at this point: How much closer can you come to the description of Jacob's ladder in Genesis 28?

As we've already mentioned, many angels in both the Old and New Testaments are presented as having a human, or humanoid appearance—and that's much the way our adventurers in immortality describe their angels. The two angels who warned Lot of the fall of Sodom in Genesis 19 are a case in point in the Old Testament. There is also every indication that the angelic messengers mentioned in the New Testament, such as those who told the first arrivals at Jesus' tomb that he had risen from the dead, were human in form.

But in some cases, as in Matthew 28:3–4, they also had a dramatic and even frightening aura about them, as the one who is described as having an "appearance . . . like lightning, and . . . raiment white as snow. And for fear of him the guards trembled and became like dead men."

There are also strange-looking angelic creatures that don't seem to appear at all in our near-death accounts. For example, the multifaced, multiwinged cherubim, which we mentioned at the beginning of this chapter, are completely absent. Also, there are the seraphim, which are referred to in Isaiah 6:2–6, and described as having six wings. They are supposed to stand next to God's throne in heaven and sing His praises there.

But even though some of these creatures don't appear in the accounts we've gathered, we recognize there are millions of stories we haven't been able to hear because of the limited sampling in our survey.

8

The Supercitizens

FROM OUR PREVIOUS DISCUSSIONS, we now have some idea about the exact identities of the beings who may possibly populate the afterlife.

Those who have had a close brush with death report in some cases the presence of a God-like figure, often identified with Christ. Angels have also played an important role in a number of people's experiences.

Finally, in still other accounts, those we've surveyed say they ran into deceased relatives. So the demographics of heaven may well be quite varied and extensive.

But now let's go in for a closer look at the bodies, minds and personalities of these deceased humans—including, perhaps eventually, some of us—who are the citizens of heaven. What exactly are these individuals like? Do they possess special powers that we don't now have? Also, do those in the afterlife experience any sort of personal growth and improvement?

As we attempt to answer these questions, we'll see that those who had a close brush with death sometimes actually experienced incredible enhancement of their spiritual, intellectual or physical powers during their encounter with immortality. In other cases, no matter what they reported happened to them personally, they at least often came away with a definite impression of what the great potential is for personal growth and transformation in the afterlife.

Now here, in more specific terms, are some of the types of personal growth reported by those who were near death, or who were temporarily dead.

A greater feeling of brotherhood and sisterhood, and of acceptance in general by others. One person who was on the verge of death because of a choking incident said she was overwhelmed by feelings of "brotherhood and acceptance." In other words, any feelings of inadequacy and lack of self-confidence may be swept away as the person moves toward heaven.

Another woman who had undergone a near-fatal auto wreck said her impression of the afterlife was, "It was wonderful. You can sit and talk to people, without any bickering going on, as we have here. There are good conversations without arguments. But that doesn't mean that for me it's an intellectually demanding experience. Some people on earth don't like to think about intellectual things—that's not the source of their happiness. I'm like that. I mean, if you have to enter into conversations where you begin to feel inferior, that's not happiness—and that's not what heaven was like for me. The intellectual part of the afterlife doesn't necessarily make any difference."

Perhaps part of the good conversation in the positive phase of the afterlife will result from what one man we interviewed described as "a sense of ministry all the time, a sense of love. In the afterlife, there is a sense of complete support and nurture among people. The interactions between individuals involve lifting one another up in every

102

way, as opposed to tearing others down. Conversations with deceased relatives are always constructive, never destructive."

In this same vein, it's interesting that 53 percent of all those we surveyed, or more than 80 million adults, said they believe that the afterlife will be characterized by "love between people."

Power over death. In a number of cases, the individual who came close to death said, "I felt I had the choice to return or not before being revived by doctors." In other cases, this idea was couched in terms of making a decision, or as one woman put it when she recalled her out-of-body state: "Soon, I would have to make a decision to stay or not. . . ."

This sense of control seems to recur again and again in the accounts we've heard. For example, one young woman from the West Coast, who nearly drowned during an accident in the ocean, said that as she began to lose consciousness, she sensed "an awareness of the reality we know on earth, but also a completely different reality. It was scary. I didn't want to leave this reality. But as I was swimming and in the process of drowning, I felt I had a choice of whether to die or not. Suddenly, it seemed as though I had become bigger than the physical forces that were threatening me!"

In a similar kind of incident, an Oklahoma woman who had undergone major surgery and almost died on the operating table "was told by God that [I] had the choice of eternal rest or continued living on earth." She chose to live when the decision was left to her, and she soon recovered from the surgery.

In a sense, this power to exist on earth or not may be analogous to what the Apostle Paul describes as the "victory over death" in the fifteenth chapter of his first letter to the church at Corinth. The idea is that death holds no more   103 fear or ultimate control over the person—he can, in effect, take it or leave it.

"Superbodies" which have special powers and are free of defects. Those who are dead and appear to relatives who are in the midst of a close brush with death have an appearance or "body" which is recognizable as the person who was once alive. But their new or heavenly bodies can do highly unusual things, such as pass through tables and closed doors, as one Illinois woman reported seeing her dead mother do as she went through a serious heart attack.

The ability to move about at will in an out-of-body condition smacks of a supermanlike quality that ordinary humans only dream about. One middle-aged woman, who came close to death after she lost a great deal of blood during childbirth, told this story: "I went into shock and could see everything going on in the room, including my own body lying on the table. I could hear everything. It was as though my spirit had left my body, and I was looking down on it."

It's interesting that even though this woman describes what we might regard as a classic out-of-body experience, she says it was *as though* her spirit had separated from her body. She is using the words that come closest to describing the experience, although the experience itself is so strange and foreign to our comprehension.

A similar kind of honest, tentative use of language occurred in the account of this Minnesota man who was undergoing treatment in an emergency room after a massive heart attack: "I felt I was lifting right out of my body. No cares, no worries, no nothing—just like I was floating. I felt I was above my body and the stretcher about four feet, just floating—a strange feeling."

Here again are some all-important words that signal the recognition that human language is not quite able to contain the extradimensional adventure: "I felt . . . just like . . . I felt . . . a strange feeling."

Finally, there is this short but dramatic account from a New Jersey woman which encompasses so many important elements of many near-death adventures in the most efficient of descriptions: "I had an accident. I was in intensive care. I saw myself going through a tunnel and saw myself lying in bed naked—my whole body just lying there in bed naked. But I felt very peaceful—no pain."

In this superbody state, the woman, despite the fact that she had been seriously injured, left her pain behind as her consciousness moved into the out-of-body condition. The tunnel sensation—which as we've seen is by no means a common, across-the-board element in the accounts of those who have been near death—may have been an extradimensional channel of some sort. In other words, as some scientists we have surveyed have speculated, it could have been a channel in space that ushered her briefly from our three-dimensional universe into a multidimensional parallel universe that constitutes the afterlife.

Also, those who have experienced a mystical kind of near-death encounter sometimes report that they have been healed of whatever infirmity was bothering them. One woman who underwent a serious stomach operation said that while she was unconscious for the first day, she took an extradimensional journey around a beautiful, unearthly landscape with strange, sparkling flowers of every color in the rainbow.

At the end of her experience, a being in a light, whom she believed was Jesus, said "You are healed." In her mystical experience, she felt healed, and the healing apparently had an impact on her physical body because when she returned to her body, she had progressed so well that the doctors sent her home the next day.

Reports of this sort agree quite well with the general

beliefs of nearly four out of ten American adults who believe that in heaven "crippled people will be whole."

Tremendous intellectual powers. People sometimes have the power to teleport themselves while lying on an operating table into an adjacent room to watch relatives waiting for the outcome of the operation. And while they observe all this happening on earth in a sort of panoramic vision, they may also be participating in some extradimensional event, such as dealing with an otherworldly being.

Nor is their perspective limited to the present. In a number of cases, people have reported to us that they had knowledge of future events as well—as the man who told us that something informed him that his mother would die by his eighteenth birthday. And sure enough, she died within a week of that time.

The total picture that we get of the enhanced mental powers is one in which thought is in no way limited by space and time. Also, thought is often integrally connected to action: The extradimensional mind "thinks," and as often as not, the extradimensional body responds. These reports from those who have been near death coincide nicely with general beliefs about intellectual and spiritual growth after death. Of the adults we surveyed, 18 percent said they felt people in heaven would grow intellectually, and 36 percent, or more than one-third of the total national sample, said they expected spiritual growth in the afterlife.

Powers of earthly senses. What we're talking about here is the ability of the individual to smell, see, hear, taste and touch things with greater awareness than would be usual. One man, for example, talked about seeing "incredible grottoes, fantastic spaces decorated with shells, organic forms. It was beautiful, exquisite, colorful, hard to describe. Like nothing I've ever seen on earth. It sounds like an hallucination when I talk about it, but it clearly wasn't for me. Also,

106

people of some sort were in the midst of all this, engaging in a festive party. The whole thing gave me a good feeling. I was experiencing and participating in this scene, as a part of the celebrating group, but I was also observing it. It was as though I was both inside of it and outside of it at the same time."

Another man, a native of North Carolina who nearly died during a heart attack, described his experience as "coming from darkness into light. There were beautiful trees and a lake with clear and beautiful water. A warm mellow glow pervaded everything, and there were no shadows, no weeds, no thorns anywhere on the landscape. The front of my body was warm, but it was pleasant, not like a hot sun."

It may not be appropriate even to refer to this kind of extradimensional encounter as using the senses, because that notion is tied too closely to the limitations of the physical body. On the other hand, those who have been close to death or have undergone related experiences and then returned, do report seeing heavenly landscapes in incredible detail, or hearing exquisite music unlike anything they have ever experienced on earth.

Control over emotions. This possible characteristic of the afterlife may be a great comfort to those who are confronting serious mental problems—and also to others who experience a periodic lack of inner peace in their lives. One man told us that a nervous breakdown he had was the worst time of his life, much worse than relatively serious physical problems. And he likened this emotional disturbance to a "hell on earth"—and probably much like the essence of the real hell itself.

But the exact opposite kind of emotional atmosphere prevails in the heavenlike dimension of the afterlife that has been reported to us. One woman who had moved from her deathbed into the presence of God and angels was fully aware of what was going on back at her hospital room, with the weeping and wailing of relatives and friends. But she wasn't emotionally disturbed by it all. It wasn't that she didn't care or that she was callous. She just seemed to be viewing everything from more of a divine perspective. Serenity, rather than turmoil, seemed to be the best description of her inner state.

In other cases, the person going through the near-death or temporary death experience may feel a sense of puzzlement as he watches the grief going on around his bedside. Or as one person put it, "I couldn't figure out why they were acting like that because I felt great, totally free of pain, as I looked down at them!"

These descriptions are reminiscent to some extent of what the New Testament calls the "peace that passes understanding." This concept has its roots in the meaning of the Hebrew term for peace, *shalom* or *salom*, but comes to full fruition in the New Testament peace concept, embodied in the Greek word *eirene*.

In the Old Testament Hebrew, *shalom* carries the connotation of completeness and well-being. It was generally used to offer a prayer for the welfare of another; to mean the state of being in harmony with another person; or to wish for the good of a city or country.

A similar kind of tranquillity of mind seems to have pervaded the emotions of many of those who had mystical near-death encounters. And in accordance with the reports of those who came close to death, the general surveys we did on attitudes and beliefs about the afterlife reveal that the most commonly accepted characteristic of the afterlife or heaven, mentioned by 65 percent of those we polled around the nation, is that "it will be peaceful."

Obedience to a higher power. The characteristics we've listed so far to describe the improvements in the personalities and bodies of those who have come close to death may lead to an assumption that they become totally autonomous and, in effect, almost all-powerful.

But such is not the case. From the Lord or other most controlling being in these visions, right down through the various angels or other creatures, a clear-cut hierarchy of authority and obedience emerges. And the dead or near-dead humans who participate in these scenes are as subject to the dictates of those above them as anyone else.

For example, in one case a man who had been near death in a hospital received a message from some sort of supernatural being. He was told that he had to travel to a faraway city for a certain purpose, and he went, without any hesitation. In other, quite typical cases, those near death or temporarily dead have followed the instructions of the Lord, a leading angel, a dead relative or other being to return to this life. Usually, the reason for the return was to care for a little child or be a companion to a spouse.

For example, one woman from Florida was involved in a terrible accident in which a seven-ton truck plowed into her car, killed her son and severely injured her. She reported that from a medical viewpoint, she had actually died and "felt lifted to a nice place," where she could see her husband back on earth praying for her. Then, she said, she felt herself "being pushed back to earth," until finally she woke up in a recovery room. Upon gaining consciousness, she cried for joy that she had been sent back to the world of the living.

In this woman's case, she apparently had little power over her ultimate return to earth, but rather was directed back here by some greater force or power. On the other hand, whether coincidentally or not, she obviously desperately wanted to live, even though she had made it to some sort of extradimensional "nice place," and her deepest wishes were realized through the work of this higher power.

A similar sort of situation involved an elderly man who was actually pronounced dead and then saw himself get out of bed and walk toward a brilliant light. But when he reached the light, some sort of person, who seemed to be in charge of things in the unearthly sphere in which the man found himself, ordered him to return to his body, and he complied.

Powers of volition, concentration or willpower. In a number of cases, the reports we received showed people in the throes of a great struggle of some sort, such as a fight to return from the vestibule or transition state of the afterlife to this world. In those cases, they show almost superhuman singleness of purpose to accomplish the task before them.

One man, for example, described an arduous crawl through an earthlike barrier to reach his body. Then, he reported, it took all the physical and mental powers of his spiritual body to accomplish the task of getting back into his physical body and getting it to work again.

⑨

The Abundant Life
in the Afterlife

SO NOW WE HAVE an idea about who may populate the afterlife, and we know something about the range of personal powers they may possess. But what are these supercitizens of heaven going to *do* with their enhanced abilities?

Those who have had a verge-of-death encounter give a variety of answers to this question, and most of the responses seem to fall into one of three main categories.

1. The citizens of heaven minister to the needs of others in heaven.

2. They minister to the needs of others on earth.

3. Finally, in addition to interpersonal ministries, they have certain jobs or duties assigned to them within the heavenly hierarchy.

1. Ministry to others in the afterlife. There is an expectation among about two out of ten American adults, as reflected in our survey on attitudes and beliefs about the afterlife, that "people will minister to the spiritual needs of others." And if the reports from those who have had a close brush with death are any indication, these beliefs are well founded.

Here is what some of those who came close to death said about the possibility of helping other deceased people.

First of all, there was a sense that we will be known thoroughly in heaven by others—in other words, they can probe our thoughts and motives and communicate with us through a form of telepathy. There will be instantaneous recognition of another person's thoughts, questions and needs.

But will those in heaven really have any needs? Or will they, by definition, be in such a state of bliss that the idea of having a need won't even exist?

Most people feel that there will be no needs in the sense of feeling inadequate or being in a state of uncomfortable deprivation. But because many feel that personal growth is possible in the afterlife, they also believe that this growth or potential for gradual improvement implies that at various points, one person may be in a position to be helped in that growth by another.

One young woman told us, "I think all our needs will be met in the afterlife and we'll be assisting each other in meeting those needs. We'll act to help one another before any needs are actually felt. It's as though a person were sitting alone, just on the verge of feeling sad or lonely, and then another person stepped in and filled the void that never quite materialized. In other words, we'll anticipate the problems of others before they actually occur and act in such perfect love that there never will be any unmet needs."

Another woman, who underwent an out-of-body experience just after experiencing the stress of a mugging, said, "I got the sense that the afterlife will involve a lot of hard work, where we'll develop our own individuality and talents in ways we've never dreamed of on earth. This may seem silly, but I actually got a message that I might be making

112

choir robes for the Archangels—mainly because I love to sew and don't get much of a chance to do that in this life. I also got the feeling that a close friend of mine, who loves working with children, will have an expanded ministry to the children of the afterlife. I really believe that in some way God is preparing many of us for our ministry in heaven through the talents we develop or feel a desire to develop here on earth."

A related impression that another person got after his near-death experience is that the friendships in heaven will be so intense that some people can help others heal feelings of jealousy, greed, selfishness or other such negative traits that may have plagued the person on earth.

Many people also used such words as "brothers and sisters," "sharers and comforters" and "guides and helpers" to describe personal relationships in the afterlife. Some of those who came near death experienced this sort of thing when a deceased relative served as their guide or instructor during the brief time they tasted eternity.

For example, one woman told us, "I, personally, was 'met' and guided along through a long dark hallway. The feeling of complete love, joy and acceptance is conveyed by everyone and everything in the afterlife. Everyone cares and looks out for each other, helping them make the transition."

Some are even convinced, after their adventure in immortality, that they will have ready access to Moses, Paul and some of the other great spiritual leaders of the past. One man told us, "I have a lot of questions about the Bible I want to ask Moses and Paul. It may be that the instant you're transformed after death that all these questions will be resolved, without your having to seek them out. But my personal feeling, after my close call with death [in a massive auto wreck in which another person was killed], is that there will be gradual growth. Perhaps we'll even be able to sit down in a heavenly lecture by some leading

113

spiritual figure—or perhaps just brainstorm one-on-one. There are so many questions I would like to talk to the people about and resolve in my mind."

Some of those who have been close to death have returned to report increased understanding after contact with a dead relative. A warm, supportive communication of this type from a dead person to one who was still living, though near death, came through in this account from a 26-year-old California man: "I was unconscious due to adverse reaction to drugs. I had taken seven drugs, and my breathing was critical. I saw myself leave the body—and also saw those working around me. And I saw my grandmother explain what had happened to me and say 'You'll live.' She had been dead for years."

As part of this spiritual learning process, one woman in our survey said she expects that all those in heaven will eventually go through every imaginable experience in a heavenly context. In her opinion, as she puts it, "sometimes you cannot learn unless you go through something yourself. I would think all people in heaven will have to go through all experiences—and that includes babies and others who die before they really become fully experienced and knowledgeable here on earth."

This woman, by the way, claimed to have spent a considerable amount of time outside her body while she was undergoing an operation. During that period, she indicates, she had extensive communications with beings who apparently started to instruct her in various spiritual matters.

Finally, another woman told us she had spent a considerable amount of time up in heaven after an operation during which she was thought to have died. As a result of this experience, she got the distinct impression that a person's ministry to others in heaven will be an extension of the kinds of work and ministry she or he had on earth. In other words, a preacher on earth would be a preacher in heaven; 114 a church usher would be some sort of usher in heaven;

and one who regularly makes hospital visits would do the same sort of thing in the afterlife.

There are obvious problems with this viewpoint if you carry it too far. For example, how can you visit the sick in hospitals if there is no sickness and there are no hospitals in heaven?

But still, an interesting aspect of this approach is that it assumes a continuity between this life and the next. In other words, just as our bodies and identities will be recognizable in the afterlife (as many in our surveys report and believe), so our special helping gifts will also carry over into the next dimension of reality.

Also, this woman believes that her experience in heaven taught her that the undeveloped parts of our own altruistic natures will be perfected as we are able to assist others in various ways. So, suppose we have neglected to give money to poor people on the streets or to lend a compassionate ear to the lonely and brokenhearted as often as we should have in this life. In that case, we'll get ample opportunity to develop those nurturing parts of our personalities in the afterlife.

These, then, are some of the ways people with near-death encounters perceived as possibilities for ministering to others in the afterlife. But what about helping people back on earth? Is that still a possibility for those who have already passed on, or is the gulf between this life and the next too great for such interaction?

2. Ministry by those in the afterlife to those who are still alive on earth. Some of the people we interviewed said flatly that they didn't believe there was any ministry or helping function that the dead could perform for the living. But others, including a number of those with a near-death experience, thought this sort of ministry was possible. And in fact, about one of every ten adults we surveyed, or about 15 million people, said they believe "one will be

115

able to minister to the spiritual needs of people on earth."

One nurse, who reported she had witnessed many death-bed scenes where the person was apparently communicating with some dead relative or another being in the afterlife, said she thinks the dead can "give us a sense of peace, security and comfort in times of trial and reflection." A number of people also said they had decided that dead relatives or friends could communicate through "dreams, visions, hunches or ESP."

Some people may object that this sort of belief borders on the occult, but the fact remains that a number of the people we talked to from some of the mainstream religious traditions said they have received this type of communication.

Others sense the possibility that contact with the dead can occur, but they don't promote it, and in fact, seem to prefer to avoid it.

One man, for instance, said, "I think that you can have contact with the dead, but most of the time I think it's satanic. Sometimes I have the sense that my great-grandmother is trying to communicate with me. She was a strong, influential person in our family—and not necessarily a positive influence."

One especially interesting interpretation of the near-death experience was the idea that some of the deceased relatives people encountered had become, in effect, guardian angels for those still alive. One person, for example, said that people in the afterlife can minister to the spiritual needs of people on earth "as comforters, guides, 'guardian angels.' "

Another said the deceased are "continually praying for those still alive, watching over them as guardian angels, maybe."

In this same vein, a middle-aged woman from the Midwest told us, "My mother is dead, and many times when a crisis arises, she tells me the right thing to do." This woman

116

actually encountered her mother during a verge-of-death experience when she was undergoing a serious operation. In that incident, the mother told the daughter to return to the "land of the living" because she (the mother) wasn't ready to receive the daughter into the afterlife just yet.

In a similar kind of encounter, a young woman, suffering from a serious injury, was pronounced dead on the operating table. "But then, I saw my mother, who had died several years before," she recalled. "She said, 'You have a daughter to raise. You have to go back!'" And in compliance with this directive, the injured woman went back and recovered from her surgery. Death, as we've seen, can be seductive because at certain points the afterlife may well begin to look more attractive than this life.

This case also seems to suggest the idea that deceased loved ones, who have a broader and more accurate perspective on our responsibilities and future prospects than we do, may sometimes step in and guide the living in more productive directions.

Another important function of heaven's citizens that several of our near-death adventurers mentioned was the idea of their serving as guides or greeters to smooth the transition from this life to the next.

On one level, the deceased may ease the process of grief that is going on among those they have left behind. One young housewife, for instance, said, "I don't know how it's done exactly, but I believe spiritual 'people' make themselves sensed or felt to comfort those they've left behind and somehow let them know they're all right. They help the survivors not to grieve their passing."

This woman said she herself was met by someone, probably her grandfather, when she was on the verge of death during a serious accident. Then she was guided into the afterlife and back by this comforting being.

Another of our respondents, a middle-aged salesman, said, "If my mother is in heaven, I think she would like to 117 guide me to be able to join her. If her mother, father, and siblings are there, she would also get them to join in together with her in helping me."

This idea of a marshaling of forces by those in heaven to have a beneficial impact on those still alive found its most dramatic expression in the observations of a schoolteacher who almost died during an appendix operation. She said, "It is difficult to define the possible ministry by those in the afterlife to the needs of those on earth. But I [have learned] that the wholeness of the spirit after life can affect those still living. I also believe the spiritual world can intervene in the daily lives of people. One could call this 'miracle work.' I believe this occurs when it is necessary for the harmony of the afterlife and the completeness of all God's purposes.

"Stopping Hitler could have been part of this process. The millions of souls in the afterlife may have finally brought their power to bear on him and his followers and ended the executions and killings of innocent human beings. Why wasn't he stopped earlier than he was? I can't answer that. But I do believe that good finally triumphed over evil because of the greater strength of God *and* of the spirits in God's presence."

This idea of helping or ministering to those who are still alive goes beyond many traditional expressions of Christian theology, though there are similarities to the Catholic idea of asking the deceased saints to pray for those who are still living. But in general, the idea of going back in some way to help those who are still wrestling with earthly problems is a point about which traditional Christian theology—and the Bible as well—are largely silent.

One passage of Scripture, which would seem to contradict the idea of a dead spirit returning to help the living, is the parable we've already mentioned in Luke 16 about the poor man Lazarus and the rich man. There, Jesus says 118 the rich man in hell asks Abraham to send back Lazarus (who is in heaven) to warn the rich man's brothers about the torments of hell. But Abraham refuses, saying, "If they do not hear Moses and the prophets, neither will they be convinced if some one should rise from the dead."

There is also a strong resistance in both the Old and New Testaments to any efforts by the living to contact the dead for help.

For example, in 1 Samuel 28, King Saul went to a woman from Endor, who was a medium, in an effort to get advice from the dead priest Samuel. The medium first objected to this procedure, but after much pressure from Saul, she finally consented. When the spirit of Samuel had been summoned, Samuel said, "Why have you disturbed me by bringing me up?" The word that Saul finally received from Samuel's spirit was equally unpleasant: Saul and his sons would be killed the next day in battle.

But despite these negative attitudes toward interaction with the dead in traditional biblical theology, there seems to be nothing that says directly that if God or one of the dead spirits wants to take the initiative and have the spirit contact the living some way, it can't be done. On the contrary, the account of Jesus at his transfiguration says that Moses and Elijah appeared on a mountain with him.

So some of the main activities of those in the afterlife will apparently have something to do with serving and ministering to others, perhaps both those who have already died and those who are still left on earth. But what about other tasks and areas of responsibilty in heaven? Are there any other work assignments that we may get when we pass over to the other side?

3. Responsibilities and duties in the heavenly hierarchy other than interpersonal ministries. We've already discussed in some detail the vestibule concept—the transition or staging area which the disembodied spirit or personality first enters before moving deeper into the extradimensional reality. Because many of the people we interviewed spent most or all of their time in this transitional place, with one

119

foot in heaven and one foot on earth, so to speak, there is really a tremendous lack of information about many aspects of what life in the afterlife may be like.

But we do have a few indications about the nature of other heavenly responsibilities from those who have come near death and then returned. For example, one lawyer who was seriously ill in a hospital said he had a sense that there would be fruit trees and other crops in the afterlife which would have to be harvested. Also, there would be vegetation, perhaps some sort of herbs, that could be used for spiritual medicinal purposes to heal the wounds and hurts, both emotional and physical, that people had suffered during their lives. This kind of healing, of course, would presuppose some sort of physican in the afterlife, a physician who might be God or an angel, but might also be a transformed human being.

Another possible area of responsibility in the afterlife that has been mentioned by those who came near death is some sort of participation in the administration or government of heaven. For example, one man told us he feels quite certain that some of those who die and go to heaven will be placed, according to their gifts and their obedience to God, at different levels in the heavenly hierarchy. They may rule over planets, solar systems or even entire universes!

The sense of physical power and tremendous intellectual and spiritual capacities of the beings that those who returned from a close brush with death have reported certainly qualify them for some kind of highly complex work or demanding leadership position. But don't get nervous and begin to think, "I'm not capable of handling the kind of global or universal responsibilities these people are talking about!" Remember: Everyone who had a heavenlike near-death experience reported feelings of emotional tranquillity and perfect control over their spiritual bodies and minds.

Some of the other work and responsibility in the afterlife, as perceived by those who had a close brush with death, is less overwhelming than this idea of being a supernatural ruler. But for many people, it's just as interesting and rewarding.

For example, one person who barely escaped from a massive auto crash said that he had the sense that "it would be possible in the afterlife to help God build His kingdom even greater, to demonstrate His power even more than has been done already. One way would be to demonstrate to the angels, who have never gone through a rebellion against God, what redemption and forgiveness by God really mean. I might be in a really strong position to help to communicate to the myriads of spirits who have never been separated from Him what His grace and love are all about—simply because I'm a fallen creature who has been restored."

These, then, are just a few of the possibilities for work, activity and responsibility in the afterlife. The reports we've received from those who have been near death are, on the whole, rather consistent with what Judeo-Christian tradition has to say on this topic—with the possible exception of the interactions some people have reported between those who have died and those who are still living.

Also, nearly two out of every ten adults we interviewed said that they believe people will have responsibilities in the afterlife.

Up to this point, we've been concentrating in minute detail on the landscape and personal characteristics of the citizens of the afterlife. But what relevance does all this information about the possible nature of the next world have for our present existence? We've put this and related questions to those who responded to our survey on near-death experiences—with some very interesting results.

10

Near Death Experiences: Afterwards

IT IS FASCINATING to contemplate the near-death incidents we've presented thus far and to speculate about what the afterlife may be like. But when you strip away the almost science-fictionlike trappings of some of the accounts and get down to the core issues that concern the average person most deeply, two major questions stand out.

1. Do these near-death accounts give those who have experienced them any reason to fear death less?

2. Is there anything about these accounts that has the power to change for the better the way a person thinks and lives his or her life?

Does the near-death experience lessen the fear of death? A rather impressive number—slightly more than one-third of those we questioned—said yes, their fear of death was lessened by their near-death encounter. Slightly less than one-third said their fear of death wasn't lessened, but at the same time, most gave no indication that their experience had aggravated their fears in any way.

When these people were questioned further about their attitudes toward death, some went into more detail about why they no longer feared death.

For example, one young woman nearly suffocated in a freak accident and during her ordeal felt herself go outside her body into an extradimensional realm that was partly in this world and partly in some other. After coming back, she reported that her views on death had definitely changed: "I did not experience any pain or fear. It seems to be an easy transition and because of my beliefs, it is a natural part of life for me to accept the idea of eternal life."

Another woman, who nearly died during an operation, was not frightened about death for herself, but did worry about her husband: "I'm not scared. I just pray that my husband will turn his life over to Christ, so that we will reign together with Him. My husband believes also that the Lord healed me. There was no other way."

After some of the anticipation of discomfort or pain often associated with death proved unfounded for an Ohio woman who came close to dying during an operation, she described her lessened fear of death this way: "Death itself is not painful. Some of the fears of death have been eliminated. Death is a phase of the life of the spirit. I have accepted death as a part of ongoing spiritual life. Death is a part of something we cannot yet understand. I believe one's death time is predetermined. We are each given a time to live and a time to die. I believe one is reunited with the spirits of loved ones at death."

A few people were so positive about their taste of death that they almost looked forward to passing away permanently! One housewife from the Midwest, who almost died during an accident and encountered one of her favorite deceased relatives during the experience, said, "I no longer have *any* fear of dying and almost envy those who pass on before me. I know where they'll be and how truly wonderful it is to be there. There is no pain or strife there. It's truly beautiful."

A number of people also found that their religious beliefs about death were confirmed or strengthened as a result of their brush with eternity. One woman who nearly died from pneumonia said flatly, "Death is not to be feared. Death is not a defeater. Christ proved it, as an example of our ongoing spirit and power."

There were also several individuals who were rather enthusiastic about the idea of dying because of the convivial companionship their near-death encounter had convinced them they would have in the afterlife. One woman said that during an extremely serious operation in which her life hung in the balance, she had met her mother and wandered around with her over a beautiful landscape filled with flowers and streams. Her conclusion after this encounter was almost euphoric: "Well, I know I will meet my father and mother and in-laws whom I loved dearly. And I am looking forward to a great reunion!"

In a number of cases, the person who had been on the verge of death made it a point to stress what a dramatic change had occurred in his attitudes. A California storekeeper who had nearly drowned on one occasion, said, "Before my experience, I was terrified of death. Now, I know that it [death] is a very peaceful feeling."

The decreased fear of death was also the result, in some instances, of the person's having been transformed during the near-death encounter from a skeptic about God to a believer. A farmer from the West Coast who met God in a blinding light during a serious operation, told us, "My views on death have changed inasmuch as I now thoroughly believe there is a presence 'out there' to receive us after death and to comfort us at the time of death."

It's been said that perhaps the most difficult aspect of death is being the one left behind. But a few people have even conquered the fear of separation and grief after their   125 close encounter with death. An Illinois woman who nearly died during a heart attack has decided, "Even the death of a loved one is a time of celebration. It is a joy to the one leaving to be in the presence of the Lord."

The lessening of the fear of death in some people is such that they have moved from relative timidity to almost an exuberant abandon in the way they live their daily lives. Far from being afraid to travel to strange places or to test unfamiliar waters, their lives are now characterized by a kind of joyous risk-taking, with little worry about the threat of death.

In this vein, a woman from the Southwest told us, "I no longer am afraid of dying or other people dying. I firmly believe there is life after this life, and therefore I'm not afraid of living this life to its fullest and even taking chances—such a free feeling!"

In fact, for some, death becomes such a nonthreatening, matter-of-fact happening that they can say, with an elderly engineer who survived a number of close calls, "I look upon death like another event and the final one in life."

Even though some people seemed almost to welcome the future possibility of their death after having had a close call, most seemed to be just as interested in living a long life, even though their fear of death had lessened. One man from the West Coast told us, "I found out that I'm not scared of death. But also, I intend to live as long as I can."

Sometimes, the near-death experience also resulted in a more philosophical, deeper view of the meaning of death. One elderly southern schoolteacher who was nearly killed during wartime said, "How close life and death are to each other. How short the walk in the parade of humanity."

These reports, then, present a rather sanguine picture of the afterlife and also an extremely encouraging picture of the outlook for eternity from a number who have tasted death and returned to tell about it. But these accounts should be kept in proper perspective. First of all, remember

126

that those who reported a definitely lessened fear of death represent a minority, even if a fairly substantial minority, of more than one-third of those we polled who said they had undergone some sort of near-death experience or the equivalent.

Also, in most of the cases involved in our study, the lives of the individuals were threatened in short illnesses, operations, or instantaneous accidents. The picture of the long, drawn-out terminal illness, in which the individual is racked by pain, doesn't emerge in these accounts.

At least one of the people we talked to who had been on the verge of death saw this point rather clearly. He said, "Dying itself is not painful. The process or means of one's death might be painful, but the cessation of life was not. The feeling that one becomes a part of something else was lasting [and positive]. Descartes's 'Cogito ergo sum'—'I think therefore I am' is pertinent here. The presence of myself in the vacuum and the presence of a 'spirit' leads me to this conclusion." (This man is referring to the fact that during his operation he sensed he was "in a great black vacuum" and saw a "presence in robes.")

As a matter of fact, most experts on death and dying will tell you that the greatest pain is in the dying process, not in death itself. And the greatest fear that an individual may have of death is actually a fear of *dying*—of being incapacitated, losing control or enduring lengthy, terminal pain—rather than the moment of death itself.

So it may be that even though these people expressed a less intense fear of death after their near-death experience, they might suffer a severe fear of dying if they suddenly found they were threatened with a drawn-out terminal illness.

Another cautionary note to keep in mind with these rather optimistic reports comes from certain theological quarters. A number of biblical scholars argue that a primary characteristic of a *personal* devil—if you happen to believe

127

in such a being—is that he is extremely manipulative and deceptive.

The argument that's made along these lines is that death is unequivocally the enemy, to be overcome only by a faith in Christ, and any reports to the contrary are nothing more than a work of satanic deception. Christian apologist C. S. Lewis has done a masterful and highly witty job of making the same point in his popular work, *The Screwtape Letters.*

But the near-death experience may affect more than just fears about the end of life; its impact may extend into a person's attitudes and activities in the present life as well. To see how this may happen, let's look at some descriptions of how the lives of those who have come close to death have been changed.

Can a near-death experience change the way a person thinks and lives in the present life? There's no doubt, from what we've been able to learn in our studies on immortality, that many of those who have been on the verge of death have returned to life with changed attitudes—attitudes that make them more positive and purposeful people.

One of the main results of many near-death incidents was a strengthening of personal religious beliefs. About 39 percent of those who had a brush with death said that their religious beliefs became stronger after the experience; 20 percent said their beliefs weren't strengthened; and another 41 percent gave no response. One man who survived a car wreck put some life into these figures by saying, "I now know, without a shadow of doubt, that God is with me every day, and God does exist. He is around all of us, everywhere."

Sometimes, the sense of inner peace and communion with God is so strong after the near-death experience that even a young person finds himself or herself looking nostalgically toward the final union with God. A young woman from Iowa told us, "I suppose I have an increased apprecia-

128

tion of life after my experience, but only insofar as I know we must be patient and wait until we're 'called home.' I know it's very wrong to take a life whether it be my own or anyone else's. But it's frustrating, especially after being there [in heaven] even for a little while." This woman, by the way, indicated that she was "definitely" sure she had seen the afterlife or heaven, and had been in the presence of God or Jesus Christ.

Along with this bolstering of inner faith, there were other ways that lives were changed. Some said they now were persuaded that God has a plan for their lives.

One elderly woman from the Midwest put it this way after a heart attack: "I have no fear of death. I just want to do what I am here for so I can one day be with the Lord and all those that are near and dear to me." Another person, an entrepreneur from California, said that his outlook on life has been changed since a near-drowning experience. He now believes that "my life here upon earth was planned and that my contributions or experiences have not yet been fulfilled."

Another way of expressing this idea of a divine plan for one's life emerged in this statement by a secretary from a Western state: "Death is not to be feared. It is the natural 'next stop' in our journey, but can be delayed with purpose or need of others—or even perhaps with appreciation and realization of our own development spiritually. I live knowing my needs will be met, with 'no thought of the morrow.' We are provided for and given the opportunity to learn and grow spiritually and get prepared for the next life. Life is more precious without the threat or fear of death."

Others mentioned a heightened perception of life's brevity and their determination to live every moment intensely. Or, as one southwestern housewife put it, "I believe in doing more things pleasing to the Lord. And I live as though every day might be my last, for I might not have another chance."

The risk-taking theme, which was mentioned earlier in this chapter, also was strong in the responses we received: Several who had undergone a mystical experience during an operation or accident said such things as, "I can even take a chance," or "It detached me, but also gave me the drive to accomplish greater things, bigger than I did before." Another way of putting this idea was that the individual had become less intimidated by the demands of life.

Also, many of those who went to the door of death said that they now have more concern for their fellow men and women. One 67-year-old woman whose mother had "called her back" when, as a young girl, she had a heart seizure, says, "It made me humble and compassionate."

Similarly, a woman who was nearly asphyxiated has become more affectionate toward others. Another, whose dead father stood beside her bed in an intensive-care ward, says she now appreciates loved ones and is more tolerant. These reactions may be best summed up in the words of an Oklahoma housewife, who concluded after a traumatic childbirth experience, "The most important lesson is that you stop and help people (all living things) by encouraging and comforting, trying to understand why people act mean and cruel. Then, you help them see that they are doing and justifying all acts from fear. It's better to do everything out of love (although I still don't always love all the time myself. . . .)"

And these inner feelings of love and concern are often manifested in concrete action. One woman became a nurse because of her experience. A man found he takes more time for his family and loved ones. A furniture salesman from the South, who feels he would have been killed in a big auto accident if he hadn't received a divine message warning him to protect himself, sums up this sort of personal change quite nicely: "I try to think about other people and the Golden Rule: 'Do unto others as you would have them do unto you.' "

Another result of a close brush with death has been heightened sensitivity to the person's place in the world around us. An elderly man from Florida is now working on his family genealogy because he has more of a sense of continuity between the past and present.

This man has also become increasingly fascinated by the natural beauty around him because of an intensification during a near-death incident of his awareness of God's creation. As a result, he says, "I now breed day lilies for fun and give away hundreds yearly."

He and a number of others who have come close to the end of life and then returned, find that their sensual perceptions of flowers, grass, sky, trees, sun and moon seem heightened beyond the awareness of those who have never looked death in the face. One individual expressed this idea in these terms: "I've learned to appreciate little things in life that we normally take for granted—like sky, trees, health, love, laughter, and most of all people's eyes!"

Another concrete result of a dramatic verge-of-death encounter was that one woman, who saw her dead father, began to "attend church more often. Also, I appreciate my loved ones more and try to be more tolerant of others."

There also is a tendency among some people to be able to "roll with the punches" of life more easily—the tragedies and disappointments that plague all of us at one time or another.

One southerner put it this way: "There are hills and valleys in life, and when I am on a hill, I look around and appreciate living that much more. When I am in a valley, I sometimes pray to God to give me strength and help me where I am weak." And because he feels that God guided him through a close brush with death, he has that much more confidence that his prayers on the more mundane matters of life will be answered.

A California designer had a similar sort of reaction after his brush with death during a serious operation. He said 131 his experience "has helped give me a detached frame of reference that maybe others might not have when adverse situations exist. But on the other hand, it gives me a drive to accomplish something greater and bigger than I would ordinarily think myself capable of—as if I must work to repay the 'second chance.' "

In a number of other cases, people who had been near death expressed a sense of balance between an increased feeling of power over themselves and their surroundings with at the same time a realistic acceptance of unalterable limitations they may have to live with.

One schoolteacher, who nearly died during an operation but found new reservoirs of inner strength in recovering his health, came to this conclusion about his abilities after the experience:

"I am less intimidated by forces which would put me in a life-or-death situation. I will not be dominated by anyone for any reason. Life is for me to live as I choose. My views give me the ability to be anyone's equal. I also believe others are my equals and should be treated as such. My life's ambitions are tempered by what I believe.

"I believe I do not have to be controlled by all outside forces. My own body determines what I can do and cannot do. I do not have to be regulated by conventional thinking. Understanding true physical and spiritual freedom makes my life a lot better."

But along with these feelings of increased power and freedom, this man said he also has learned to accept difficult situations more easily since his brush with death. "Practicing freedom is constant and ongoing. Sometimes I have to remind myself to practice it when life gets thorny. But I find I can accept more things I have no control over. I can lead my daily life accepting its difficulties easier now. I have health problems which are bearable. I know there are things not meant for me to understand yet. I know at some point my spirit will at last know, understand and accept."

For the most part, those who have undergone a near-death incident which was accompanied by some unusual mystical encounter, feel that they are better people for the experience. One lawyer told us, "I have more inner peace. I tend, more and more, to leave things to my Lord—especially things I could really muck up if I muddled about with it. I don't push the panic button as often or as hard."

A New Jersey housewife had a similar kind of impression as she pondered her brush with death. "I enjoy life more, and I try not to let things worry me as much. I pray about them and ask the Lord to help me work them out."

This sense of inner tranquillity and proper spiritual proportion for things has also affected her attitude toward her possessions: "Material things don't worry me like they used to. They wear out. God's love never wears out."

Despite the fact that she almost lost her life in an operation, this woman has concluded, "It was so beautiful. All I went through was worth the experience I was with the Lord and enjoyed being in His presence. I knew He loved me so much. I knew He loved me before, but felt it more with my [operation and] healing."

Finally, there is a kind of physical courage that comes out in a few of the accounts that we received. This is something that goes beyond mere risk-taking for one's own ambitions in life, but rather focuses on sacrifice for others. One Indiana psychologist, who nearly died in a freak accident around her home, expressed this thought beautifully:

"You realize and appreciate how easy it is to be alive one moment and dead the next. I am not really afraid of death. I only don't want to die because I have too much to do on earth and it would cause a lot of pain for family and friends. I would rather be one of the last to die so I don't cause too much pain for others."

This statement is worth reading again and meditating upon. What many of us tend to fear most is losing a loved one, not losing our own life. The idea of being one of the 133 last survivors of a family—being alone and perhaps incapacitated at an advanced age—may be a more fearful prospect than dying quickly and painlessly in the prime of life.

So this woman, after her near-death event, had acquired what she regarded as a sufficiently intimate knowledge of God and the afterlife for her to be willing to say, in effect, "I'm now ready to put up with the grief and loneliness of being the last to die—because I *know* what the future life holds for me!"

On the whole, then, there are many positive changes that have occurred in the attitudes and actions of those who have come close to death and then returned to tell about it.

11

The Twilight Zone

THERE ARE CERTAIN AREAS of study, belief and fantasy that have burgeoned—especially in the United States—in the last two decades and that might be lumped under the general terms "paranormal," "quasi-spiritual" or "popular scientific speculation."

Some of the key notions that may be associated with these lines of thought are a belief in contact with the dead, extraterrestrial life, reincarnation, and supermental powers like ESP (extrasensory perception).

Now admittedly, concepts like those mentioned above are by no means synonymous with one another. In fact, they may represent quite different lines of thought and spiritual or intellectual discipline. Also, people who believe in one may be horrified at the thought that anyone might assume that they believe in any of the others. Many people who believe in ESP do not believe it is possible to have contact with the spirits of dead people.

But even though there are significant differences between these unusual beliefs, they frequently have certain key elements in common. One of these elements may be a belief that our destiny, either as individuals or as a species, is capable of being influenced or controlled from some source either outside our own human community or outside our traditional religious sources of spiritual authority.

Another common thread that runs through this line of thinking is that part or all of the ultimate truth and understanding of the universe may lie in somewhat strange, largely unknown areas of inquiry. Not everyone who holds one of these speculative views necessarily makes either or both of these assumptions. But many people do, and the result may be a strong spiritual challenge to traditional religious faith as these notions capture the attention, imagination and sometimes even the ultimate allegiance of those who get involved.

The special relevance of this subject matter to our present study of near-death experiences is that both deal with a kind of spiritual frontier, a twilight zone of belief and speculative inquiry. But what are the similarities and what are the differences between these two areas of thought and experience? To find out, let's look more closely at some of the speculative beliefs in our society and try to understand how they may be distinguished from, or related to, what we've learned about those who have come close to death.

The first important step is to get an overview of the range of unusual beliefs that people may hold. In a recent study we conducted on beliefs in the occult, supernatural beings and various paranormal phenomena, we found the following beliefs among adult Americans.

• A solid majority (or 57 percent) of adult Americans aware of UFOs (unidentified flying objects) believe that they are real. This figure contrasts markedly with Great Britain, where only 27 percent said they believe in flying saucers.

• Slightly more than half of those polled in the general

American population believe in ESP, but the figure rises to nearly two-thirds for those people with a college background.

In our most recent study, conducted especially for this book, we concentrated on just three main areas of belief in this speculative area: 1) reincarnation; 2) extraterrestrial life; and 3) contact with the dead. In the general population, we discovered that quite a large minority of people hold these beliefs, with an especially heavy expression of conviction among young people and those who live on the West Coast.

For example, take reincarnation, or the rebirth of the soul in a new body after death. Of those adults we polled, 23 percent, or nearly one-quarter, said they believe in reincarnation.

The belief in reincarnation rises to 27 percent among those who live in the West and drops to 16 percent among those who live in the Deep South. A possible reason for this regional variation may be that the West Coast is more susceptible to the influence of Eastern religions, which include reincarnation as an article of faith. In the Deep South, on the other hand, evangelical Christianity has a much stronger hold than in some other parts of the country, and reincarnation is anathema to traditional New Testament doctrine. However, southern blacks show an especially high belief in reincarnation, with 32 percent replying "yes" in our survey.

There is also a significant variation among age groups as far as reincarnation is concerned. Nearly one-third (30 percent) of those 18 to 24 years old said they believe in reincarnation. But that figure goes down steadily as older people are asked about their beliefs: When you reach the 50 and older group, only 21 percent express a conviction that reincarnation actually occurs.

Involvement in organized religion also seems to have

a strong impact on this belief. About 17 percent of those we surveyed who attend church regularly said they believe in reincarnation, while 27 percent of those who don't attend regularly believe. This may be an indication that those who are going to church regularly are more likely to hear and believe traditional Christian doctrine, which denies reincarnation, than are those who rarely or never darken a church door.

There are a number of similarities, but also some clear-cut differences, between these responses to our question about reincarnation and another question we asked about extraterrestrial life. We asked, "Do you believe there is human life on other planets or not?" and a resounding 46 percent of the general population replied "yes," they believe there is.

There were far more (54 percent) of those from the West who believed in extraterrestrial life than those in the Deep South (30 percent). Also, age played an important role in this belief, with 55 percent of those under 30 saying that they believe there is life on other planets, and only 38 percent of adults over 50 saying they believe.

Also, there was a significant difference between Protestant and Catholic beliefs on this subject. Nearly 52 percent of Catholics expressed a belief in life on other planets, while less than 43 percent of Protestants hold the same conviction. In addition, more men than women believe in extraterrestrial life, by 50 percent to 43 percent.

Finally, there is a dramatic correlation between traditional religious beliefs and church involvement, and a lack of belief in life on other planets. Only 37 percent of those who attend church regularly said they believe there is extraterrestrial life, while nearly 52 percent of those who don't attend believe. Also, only 40 percent of those who say religion is "very important" in their lives affirm this belief, while more than 56 percent of those who say religion is "not very important" believe in extraterrestrial life.

This disparity on the basis of religious involvement may be the result of the following factors. First of all, some people with a scientific bent, as we'll see in a later chapter, tend to reject traditional religious concepts. As a result, they have no reason to regard human life as unique or necessarily limited to this earth, and they may move naturally toward a belief in life on other planets through scientific or logical analysis.

But at the same time, there may well be a substantial number of people outside the traditional religions who are casting about for meaning in life. As a result, they may embrace a concept like extraterrestrial beings who possess special knowledge and skills that could help us "inferior" earthlings improve our lives. For some people, the spacemen may even become a kind of religious substitute. Some popular movies, like *Close Encounters of the Third Kind,* reflect such a response.

The third main speculative area that we focused on in our latest survey was the possibility of contacting the dead. Specifically, we asked, "Do you think it is possible to have contact with the dead or not?"

A substantial number of adult Americans take this topic very seriously. In the general population, about a quarter (24 percent), or perhaps 37 million people, believe it is possible to contact the dead.

The geographical pattern that we have seen developing with respect to other unusual beliefs also applies in the case of a belief in contact with the dead. One in three adults in the West believe, while only two in ten of those in the South do.

Also, there is a startling difference in beliefs on this subject among the different age groups, with a pattern from more to less belief emerging as people get older. An amazing 38 percent of young adults under 30 say they believe it's possible to contact the dead, while only 12 percent of those 50 years old or older have this conviction.

In addition, our study shows that church and religious involvement also have an impact on this belief. Only 18 percent of those who attend church regularly said they believe it's possible to contact the dead, while a significantly higher 27 percent of those who don't attend church have this conviction. Also, 21 percent of those people who said that religion was "very important" in their lives stated that they believe in the reality of contact with the dead. In contrast, the percentage of those who believe climbed to 27 percent among people who say religion is not very important.

As is the case with beliefs in reincarnation, it may be that those who are deeply involved in traditional religion are more likely to be imbued with the orthodox doctrine and thus less likely to affirm a belief like the possibility of contact with the dead. You'll recall that we discussed in another context how there is a strong resistance in both the Old and New Testaments to summoning up deceased spirits.

What relationship do these paranormal and speculative beliefs have to our reports about near-death experiences?

First of all, there is some overlap between those who affirm these beliefs and those who have had a close brush with death.

For example, one young New York housewife who responded to our near-death survey said, "I believe in reincarnation—that as good a life as you try to live now, your next life will be as good or better. Likewise, if your life now centers on malice and self-centeredness, your next life will probably be worse to you." This woman also told us that she believes it is possible to have contact with the dead.

Her near-death experience, however, was not as otherworldly as some of the others related to us. She underwent a close call with drowning during a boating accident on some dangerous rapids. As she went under for what might

140

have been the last time, she prayed to God. She then recalls, "Fortunately the water became shallower, and I was able to cling to a rock until my friends could reach me."

But in her case, there was no particularly unusual mystical encounter. She said she did not feel she had a glimpse of an afterlife or heaven. She did feel she might have been in the presence of God or Jesus Christ—perhaps as a result of the prayer she offered. But her belief in reincarnation seems to have had no connection with her near-death experience.

There are also some reports of encounters with dead people apart from any near-death experiences described in our near-death surveys. One example that we've already considered in another context bears repeating at this point. In a direct, firsthand report of this sort, a middle-aged housewife from the East Coast first described her own brushes with death:

"Twice, in very close calls in automobile accidents, I have had a vivid experience of my life literally rolling backwards before my eyes at a great speed.

"Also, while undergoing a Caesarean section under emergency circumstances and being in very poor physical condition, I had an experience of being in the room with myself, but standing apart from everything going on. I did not care what happened, and felt that it was very unimportant."

This housewife, like the one in the boating accident, believes in reincarnation as well as in contact with the dead. And these convictions put them with a substantial number of other people who have had both near-death experiences and hold one or more of the paranormal or speculative beliefs.

In this regard, our findings reveal that of those who have been on the verge of death, 31 percent believe in reincarnation, as opposed to 23 percent of the general public. Secondly, 54 percent of those who have faced death   141 believe there is life on other planets, in contrast to 46 percent of the general public. Finally, 31 percent of those who have come close to death believe it's possible to contact the dead, as compared with about 24 percent of the general public who believe.

What these figures suggest is that there is a consistent correlation between a near-death experience and a relatively high belief in paranormal or other unusual phenomena. One possible explanation for this correlation may be that an encounter with what seems to be the afterlife in a verge-of-death incident tends to open up the person to a consideration of other types of unusual, extra-ordinary experiences. A high percentage of scientists in our society carry this connection one step further and argue that those who think they have had mystical near-death experiences or accept as valid such speculative notions as reincarnation or contact with the dead are deluded. To understand the scientific and medical contentions more fully, let's now turn to a consideration of what the scientists and physicians we've interviewed have to say.

12

What Does Science Have to Say?

BY POPULAR TRADITION, scientists are a tough-minded, skeptical lot, not at all inclined toward belief in spiritual or supernatural matters. If you can't touch it, analyze it or put it in a test tube, it's not real or worth considering further.

But is this common image a reflection of what scientists are actually like?

Our surveys and interviews with a representative sampling of medical doctors and other scientists from Marquis's *Who's Who in America* reveal that there is, indeed, an element of truth in the stereotype. This group tended to be much less inclined to believe in religious concepts, such as the afterlife, than people in the general national polls we conducted. And they are almost overwhelmingly skeptical about the validity of the near-death accounts—at least, insofar as those accounts purport to open windows on an objective supernatural or extradimensional reality.

To get a complete picture of where these physicians and other scientists stand on various spiritual matters, let's first take a look at their general beliefs on a variety of supernatural subjects. Then we'll delve more deeply into their opinions and interpretations, both positive and negative, of the near-death encounters we've been discussing.

We divided our survey equally between medical doctors and scientists who specialize in other disciplines. Because there are significant variations in the way that these two groups view spiritual matters, we'll be discussing them separately under the labels "physicians" and "scientists" as we go along. As is our custom in national surveys of this type, we'll report the opinions of these individuals in their own words, but without revealing their names or specific identities.

Only 16 percent of the scientists we surveyed said they believe in life after death. On the other hand, that figure jumps to 32 percent, or about one-third, of the physicians we polled. But both these results are far below the two-thirds, or 67 percent, of the general public who say they believe in life after death.

A very low four percent of scientists say they believe in hell, while 15 percent of the physicians have this conviction. These levels of belief, of course, are far below the 53 percent of the general adult public that believe in hell.

The pattern continued when we asked these two groups "Do you think there is a heaven, where people who have led good lives are eternally rewarded?" A low eight percent of the scientists answered "yes," and 24 percent of the physicians replied in the affirmative. In our survey of the general public, on the other hand, 71 percent of all adult Americans said they believe in heaven.

As far as some of the unusual or paranormal beliefs are concerned, these two scientifically oriented groups, once again, had far fewer believers than the general population. Only eight percent of the scientists believe in reincarnation, and a comparable nine percent of physicians have this conviction. These figures are well below the 23 percent of the general population who believe in reincarnation.

144   As for contact with the dead, five percent of the scientists

said they believe and nine percent of the physicians affirm this conviction. In the general public, in contrast, 24 percent think it's possible to get in touch with those who are deceased.

Finally, there are more believers among scientists than physicians as far as human life on other planets is concerned. A strong 35 percent of the scientists responded that they do believe there is life on other planets, while 25 percent of the physicians believe. As for the general public, 46 percent are believers on this particular issue.

Why should the beliefs of these two groups jump up so dramatically on this point, and yet stay quite low on all the others? Probably because there is a sense among a substantial minority of the scientifically trained community that, with such a large number of solar systems in the universe, life similar to ours may have evolved. This is a conviction based on logical analysis of odds and probabilities, not on faith, so it's easier for a scientist to hold such a position.

Scientists and physicians often begin with a bias of disbelief. That's important to keep in mind as we discuss their approach to near-death incidents.

Of course, there may well have been biases built into the accounts we've received of verge-of-death experiences. For example, 67 percent of those who have had a close encounter with death believe in life after death, and 71 percent of these people believe in heaven. What we don't know is how many of these people believed in the afterlife, heaven or other spiritual things before their near-death experience, and how many became believers as a result of the experience.

We do know that 39 percent of those who came close to death had their religious beliefs strengthened as a result of the experience. But the chances are, many more of them were likely to have been believers in some sort of spiritual realm before their experience than the average scientist or physician.

So, the views of scientists and physicians are extremely

valuable in helping us get a proper perspective on the many near-death incidents we've uncovered.

First of all, we asked these scientifically oriented groups the same personal question we put to the general public: "Here is a question about unusual experiences people say they have had when they have been on the verge of death or have had a 'close call'—such as experiences of continued life or an awareness after death. Have you, yourself, ever been on the verge of death or had a close call which involved any unusual experience at that time?"

It's important to note here, by the way, that none of the physicians and scientists we'll be quoting knew about the specific studies we've done for this book. On the other hand, all who responded were aware in general of the phenomenon of the near-death encounter, either as a result of other books, press accounts or their own personal experiences.

We found that ten percent of the scientists and nine percent of the physicians said they had a verge-of-death experience—as compared with 15 percent of the general public.

These close encounters with death had some impact on their beliefs, as they did on the beliefs of those in the general public. For example, more than half the scientists and slightly less than half of the physicians said that the experience had lessened their fear of death. Also, a quarter of the scientists and a comparable number of physicians reported that their religious beliefs had been strengthened after their near-death incident.

How do the representatives of these groups—whether they have had a close call or not—tend to interpret their experiences?

The key question we asked of all these people was, "As you know, people who have been on the verge of death or have had a very close call, sometimes report having what are described as 'near-death experiences.' These can include 'out-of-body' experiences and experiences that are some-

146

times perceived to be a relevation of another dimension of the universe or a revelation of God. How do you, yourself, assess these experiences?"

First of all, let's take some of the positive responses, which represent a small minority of those we questioned. It should be noted, by the way, that almost all those who replied affirmatively said they also believe in a life after death, and this may have had a significant influence on their answers.

One scientist told us, "Repeated instances have been reported under scientific observation within the medical community of body-soul separation for varied periods of time. The victim has been able to accurately recall and account for many minute details that occurred in the room after having been pronounced 'dead.' But then life has been resumed under the care of competent professional personnel. Some of my personal experiences, studies, etc., would have me believe that such reports from reliable sources are not beyond the realm of possibility."

Another positive assessment came from a California research physicist, who has himself had some near-death mystical experiences: "I have had personal experiences along these lines which only increase my introspection and various hypotheses—though not my actual knowledge. Several times during a reputably severe illness, I have seen strangers walk through my room, coming from physically impossible locations. Several times, my arms and hands were detached from my body, yet were under my full control. They could go where I wished and at my bidding. All these experiences were pleasant."

Some of the other positive responses from scientists were much more terse: "I believe they are real." "I believe them to be 'real,' i.e., contact with another dimension." "They are real and true."

But with characteristic scientific caution, others could give only a qualified nod to the validity of the near-death accounts. A medical researcher in virus diseases, for exam- 147 ple, said, "They could be real. I wouldn't discount these experiences. Of course, they could just be a dream. However, since no one has proven it, I choose to believe that these experiences are real."

One specialist in surgical oneology said, "They may be true, but so far, to my knowledge, they have been momentary and inconclusive."

These positive or neutral answers are in a distinct minority, however. By far, the largest number of in-depth interpretations we received from scientists and physicians were intended to show that the near-death accounts were *not* connected with the afterlife or an extradimensional realm of reality.

Even those who themselves had had an unusual near-death experience sometimes refused to accept it as being explainable in other than scientific terms. For example, an academic physician from Florida told us he had "rolled over in a car 30 years ago, and my life 'flashed before me.' I didn't see God, but I was out-of-body."

He explains his own sensations, as well as those of others in similar situations, as a "phenomenally heightened awareness, endorphins [a hormonal substance that acts like morphine when released under stress or heavy exercise in the human system], and the perspicacity of the survivor."

Another typical kind of response came from one physician who said he does believe in life after death, though not in the objective reality of near-death reports. He stressed the fact that many of those in some reports hadn't really died (despite the reports of a few of our respondents that they had been *declared* dead).

"These are undoubtedly cerebral manifestations which the subject recalls. The individual has not died in the episode as is evident by his or her return to consciousness, and cerebral activity has *not* ceased (no 'brain death'). This is evidenced by the subject's relating of his impression. Such cerebral manifestations are completely possible and logical.

148

Content [of the visions, etc.] is determined by the individual's past and present beliefs, attitudes, wishes, etc., as in dreams."

Brain death, as we've mentioned in another context, is a medical concept in which a cessation of brain waves, along with certain other criteria, are used to show that the person is actually dead.

Many of the other responses we received differed slightly in shades of meaning and interpretation. But most came down to the basic conclusion that the trauma of a near-death experience triggered something in the brain that made it only seem as though the person was really entering another dimension. In fact, these scientists and physicians believe, everything the person is "seeing," "hearing," or "doing" in this reality is actually just going on in his mind. Listen to what some of them say:

• A Maryland biophysicist: "These are the experiences of a mind in an abnormal state physiologically, where many of these people believed that they had already died. The brain is a very complex organ and it can play a lot of tricks when you mistreat it—look at the experiences with hallucinogenic drugs."

• A geologist from California: "They could be the biochemical and electrical discharge or relaxation of the brain—that is, the barely conscious manifestations of such discharge. If so, then any combination of all past memory and/or imagination would be possible. The fear or anticipation of death could easily channel such a process, thus increasing the frequency of similar imagery among a large population beyond random probability."

• A scientist from the West Coast: "These are dreamlike states, triggered by random nerve firings, but running their course in a context of preestablished beliefs and expectations."

This man, by the way, reported an unusual near-death   149

experience himself. He said, "As I was being etherized for a tonsillectomy, I felt myself detaching from my body on the operating table and rotating around it. This state lasted for four to five seconds at most." He doesn't believe in life after death and doesn't think the out-of-body sensation had any element of objective reality about it. It just happened in his mind.

• An Ohio psychiatrist also was highly skeptical about the whole subject: "I feel that these reports are fantasies or hallucinatory phenomena. The reports are consistent with prior information and opinions. Also, these reports can be duplicated by magicians."

• A professor of pharmacology told us: "These experiences are most probably attributable to derangements of brain function in some patients near death, caused either by oxygen deficiency, drugs or products of faulty metabolism, and are essentially not different from the so-called 'psychedelic trip' elicited by LSD or other psychoactive drugs or poisons. The classical description of such an experience was given by the great American physician Oliver Wendell Holmes in a self-experiment with ethyl ether, and I quote, in part, 'The mighty music of the triumphal march into nothingness reverberated through my brain, and filled me with a sense of infinite possibilities, which made me an archangel for the moment. The veil of eternity was lifted. The one great truth which underlies all human experience, and is the key to all the mysteries that philosophy has sought in vain to solve, flashed on me in a sudden revelation. Henceforth all was clear; a few words had lifted my intelligence to the level of the knowledge of the cherubim. As my natural condition returned, I remembered my resolution; and staggering to my desk, I wrote, in ill-shaped, straggling characters, the all-embracing truth still glimmering in my consicousness. The words were these . . . A strong smell of turpentine prevails throughout.' "

150   • A professor of surgery from Iowa: "These are flash re-

calls based on a sudden surge (limited) of excitation of brain cells. This occurs many times without 'close call' experiences when one suddenly has a memory recall at an unexpected moment. The temporary restriction of circulation or oxygen supply to brain cells (as in near death) is followed by a rebound hyperemia and an increase in the stimulus to the brain's memory banks.

"The individual after the fact perceives the extraordinary experience as 'divine or out of this world.' These are difficult to prove or disprove, but as a rational man, I [can] think of other explanations."

• A 73-year-old specialist in internal medicine from Texas: "Most of these have not been really 'near-death,' and when they are, the experiences are psychoneurotic, imagined or expected on the basis of belief. Few if any of the many dying I have seen have had other than delirium, including some who have staged partial recovery."

• A New York physician who believes in the afterlife was nevertheless similarly negative in his assessment. "They are very sincere, but usually the descriptions are plagiarized or borrowed from others."

• A Pennsylvania surgeon with a somewhat psychoanalytic interpretation: "These experiences are hallucinations based upon stories, legends and beliefs of parents, etc. The ideas of lights, ghostly figures, religious symbols, etc., are firmly implanted into the minds of most children at an early age, and perhaps the brain releases them under such stress."

• One interesting tie-in with the joggers' "high" that sometimes occurs after running several miles came from a specialist in internal medicine from Maryland: "Physical state can affect mental perception. On a much lesser scale, some who enjoy jogging find they have new insights or think more clearly or along new avenues while running."

(Recent research has shown, by the way, that running may also release those endorphins, or morphinelike hor-   151 mones, that can give a feeling of well-being and otherwise affect the mental capacities of the individual.)

• Fear of death was an important element seen by a medical professor specializing in clinical pharmacology, anesthesia and physiology: "They are simply hallucinatory and based on fear of death. They occur during an altered physiologic state of the brain."

• A psychiatrist from California put an almost exclusive stress on the psychological aspects of the experience: "It's wish fulfillment," he said.

• A professor of chemistry stressed that injured brains do not provide a reliable basis for reporting any sort of experience: "My guess is that they are related to dreams or hallucinations. Of all the perceptions or revelations attributed to humans, those that are most trustworthy have come from the best brains in the healthiest conditions. A brain that has been in shock or deprived of oxygen as one near death is hardly in the best condition. Further, I have been near death a number of times—once unconscious for eight hours, once through electrically induced cardiac arrest followed by resuscitation. These experiences were simply like restful, dreamless sleep."

• One of the most interesting chemically oriented explanations we received came from a chemical physicist from Iowa: "These are likely a manifestation of the biochemistry of the brain which has become oxygen deficient during these episodes. Also, the hormonal system is likely to change, thereby producing hallucinations.

"These reported experiences differ little from those given by those under the influence of drugs, such as LSD. The body can produce similar altered states, e.g., the runner's high. Thus, such feelings on return from the threshold of death may be expected. They may be nature's defense from the terror of death. After all, it is something nature must have evolved as a defense."

• A neuroscientist from New York has decided that the

near-death accounts are merely an example of how people use known concepts in their lives to interpret entirely new experiences: "Near-death experiences constitute a set of sensory and perceptual stimuli which are entirely new to the individual. We tend to mold new experiences into some format which 'fits' other experiences we have had. We reinterpret new experience to fit long-held beliefs. If one believes in the 'supernormal,' then one will distort a unique new experience in terms of these beliefs. Such experiences (near-death) do not 'prove' the existence of 'life after death' or 'God' or whatever, but confirm the ease and variety of interpretations given new experiences."

• One nuclear scientist focused on a comparison of the near-death reports with what he knows about dreams: "People, when asleep, often have very specific categories of dreams (flying, falling, running away while rooted to the ground, etc.). Point-of-death dreams, like other categories of dreams, have their similar features because of the similarities in human mental responses."

• A New Jersey neurologist who specializes in cases involving the issue of brain death: "[These experiences are] in accordance with what we know about anesthesiology."

• A specialist in clinical pathology from Virginia: "Probably these cases are biological phenomena—related to daydreaming in a brain being deprived of oxygen and glucose at a certain rate or in a certain sequence."

• A similar kind of explanation came from a Wisconsin ophthamologist: "These experiences demonstrate the effects of anoxia [a deficiency of oxygen reaching body tissues] and/or various 'flight and fright' hormones on the brain."

• A Michigan scientist: "These are trauma-induced fantasies. Dreams often deal with the anxieties of the time, so death anxiety leads to death-associated fantasy."

• One of the more complex explanations came from a molecular biologist based in New York: "The near-death experiences are reconstructions by the brain based on accu-

153

mulated sensory inputs and an acute focus on the current state as seen in an unencumbered (from exterior inputs) reference frame."

• A specific knowledge of some of the other literature in this field came through in this response from one of our New Jersey respondents: "The reports of [Elizabeth] Kubler-Ross, [Dr. Raymond] Moody and others are exceedingly interesting, but in need of replication and extension. Studies so far are very unsystematic. The findings are subject to alternative explanations, such as common biochemical and psychological properties. Alternatives to the easy hypothesis—common experiences suggest the existence of God and an afterlife—have not been ruled out."

• A chemical physicist from New York had this to say: "Our living body functions much like a continuous flow chemical reactor with parallel paths, which are in dynamic equilibrium. A temporary halt along one path need not cause immediate, total collapse if another path can assume the functions of the disrupted line through a temporary overload. Such a drastic change *is* a revelation of God, who designed life."

But this chemist indicated that he doesn't believe in the afterlife. He told us, "Physical life after death of a human being as the *same* human being cannot continue after death, or there would be no death. However, one's issue will live on as different human beings, bearing some of one's characteristics, and the body's organic matter will help support new life. One's reputation can live on, essentially forever, in the memory of future generations."

• A Pennsylvania physicist touched on a specific aspect of the near-death experiences: "I assume that 'near-death experiences' are a part of dying. That can include 'out-of-body' experiences. But it is nonsense to interpret them as 'real.' They just happen in the minds of these dying people."

• A Massachusetts psychiatrist was more or less noncommittal about his own position—but not about what he perceives as the view of the general population: "I see people every day in my psychiatric practice who believe in such things, but 90 percent of the population will argue they are crazy."

• Perhaps the best summary of the position of the non-believers came from this Texas engineer: "The human mind is a complex and wonderful thing, whose full range of capabilities are not yet within our ability to understand. The 'experiences' are not real." In other words, the brain is doing something incredible in these near-death experiences, but everything is occurring *inside* the brain only, not in any outside, objective reality.

• On the other hand, a Ohio biologist regarded the experiences as real, but with an important qualification: "I believe them to be real, but I do not necessarily look upon them as a revelation of God or another dimension of the universe. The stories related are too 'earthly' or represent experiences believed or beliefs or concepts of heaven, hell or other worlds."

Some of the scientists and physicians we contacted became so agitated by our questions about near-death experiences that they responded almost belligerently: "Bosh! . . . Complete hogwash! . . . Journalistic fiction or delusions! . . . Hokum, baloney, nonsense. . . ."

A gerontologist went even further when we asked if he had had a near-death experience: "I haven't but I can't resist inventing an answer—so here goes: I was floating on a fluffy cloud in bright sunshine and knew that for the first time in my life I didn't have to worry about getting sunburned. Then, I tried out my wings and flew all around heaven. Then, Jesus Christ kissed me, and told me I had won the Jehovah Prize which was a bigger honor than the Nobel Prize. Then, I noticed that I was whole again—my gallbladder had grown back and my pimples disappeared."

A more thoughtful response came from a geologist and 155

paleontologist who believes that the near-death accounts are hallucinations. But he said, "I do believe there is evidence for telepathic communications between living individuals, and that demonstration thereof, in a scientific sense, may someday become available."

This man went on to describe the basis for his belief: some personal experiences with telepathy which come close to a number of our near-death accounts. He said, "I have observed demonstrable evidence for a communication between a man and his daughter (my wife), at a distance of several thousand miles at the time, just prior to the death of the father. The father said, in effect, 'Good-bye.' One friend of mine has told me a comparable experience of his, where the two people involved were mentally and emotionally known to be very close."

Another scientist found himself probing in a similar intellectual direction: "I believe they are unusual, human psychological phenomena, resulting from mental processes we do not understand (e.g., ESP)."

Perhaps it's best to end these interpretations by scientists and physicians on the gracious and thoughtful note struck by this scientist from Iowa:

"To the person to whom these experiences occur, they are very real. Their response to them is somewhat conditioned by their religious attitudes. For one, it may be considered as God revealing himself in some way to that person. To another, it may be a psychological phenomenon within the person. My personal belief is that God can and does intervene in some instances—the difficulty is determining what is a legitimate God experience."

13

The Clergy and the Close Call

IN THIS BOOK, we've been dealing with concrete accounts that purport to be eyewitness reports of an eternal, supernatural dimension of reality. At various points, we've compared the empirical evidence we've gathered with various traditional religious viewpoints. And, as we've seen, some aspects of the near-death encounters tend to support traditional religious explanations of the afterlife, while other aspects go well beyond any particular system of belief.

This is not to say that what we've found conflicts with or contradicts ideas of immortality that have sprung up from the Judeo-Christian tradition—just that the reports of those who have been at death's door and returned may provide a considerably expanded picture of what the afterlife is all about.

But so far, our comparison of the "evidence" of the afterlife and the "official" religious views has been rather piecemeal. Now, let's explore in more detail how our findings stack up against several classic religious expressions of the nature of the afterlife.

For this comparison, we'll examine four main religious traditions that seem most relevant to the findings that we've uncovered—evangelical Christian, traditional Roman Catholic, liberal Protestant and Catholic, and several approaches in Judaism. We won't consider any of the non-Western religions, because, perhaps because of the demographics of our surveys or for some other reason, there is relatively little correlation between their views of the afterlife and our specific near-death reports.

1. Evangelical Christian. The term "evangelical Christian" is a catchall phrase which includes many traditions in both the Protestant and Catholic churches. It may include those who claim to be born-again—and according to various surveys we've done, as many as 50 million adult Americans say they have had such a clearly identifiable Christian conversion experience.

The term evangelical Christian may also be defined more restrictively to include those who say they 1) have had a born-again experience; 2) have tried to encourage someone else to accept Jesus Christ as his or her savior; and 3) accept the Bible as the actual word of God, to be interpreted literally, word for word. We have found that about 30 million adult Americans are evangelical Christians in this second, more restrictive sense. Of these, 87 percent were Protestant, 12 percent were Catholic and one percent were Jewish (apparently Jewish Christians or "messianic Jews").

Because all evangelicals tend to take the Bible very seriously as their primary source of spiritual authority, their views on all religious matters—including heaven, hell and the afterlife—are influenced decisively by what the Scriptures say. But as with many other subjects, the answer to the question of what life after death is really like can get extremely complex, even when a person accepts what the Bible says as completely true and accurate.

The reason for this is that the landscape and the population of heaven and hell are not clearly described in minute detail in any one section of the Scriptures. To the contrary, there are numerous suggestions, hints and indirect references to the afterlife which must be studied and pulled together in some fashion to get as complete a picture as possible. And because even people with a similar theological orientation will not always draw the same inferences from any given set of biblical suggestions or facts, there are many different views about precisely what the afterlife may be like.

Similarly, when it comes to the question of the meaning of the near-death experiences we have been discussing, there is a difference of opinion. Some would say, with many scientists, that these incidents are nothing more than the figments of people's imaginations. Others would say they are satanic ruses to distract human beings from God's true will and purposes. Still others, who take the Bible just as seriously, would allow for the possibility that at least some of these mystical experiences, which are reported in connection with close brushes with death, provide a true window on immortality.

For example, evangelist Billy Graham at one point seems to have left open the possibility that there may be some justification for regarding near-death experiences as a kind of window on the afterlife. He told us, "Dr. Raymond Moody has interviewed more than one hundred people who have medically died and come back to life. He has put these intervews in a bestseller entitled *Life After Life,* which comes the closest to illustrating what it is like to die. Still, it is not an easy thing for people to describe. Often, they stutter and fall silent, faced with the unconceivable task of telling something which is beyond earthly experience."

A more negative explanation is offered by Bible scholar Charles Ryrie. In discussing earlier studies, especially those by Dr. Raymond Moody, Ryrie says: "There probably is no single answer that would apply to all cases. It is clear   159 that in no case was the person dead in the total sense of the concept. It is clear that similar experiences can be induced psychologically in healthy persons; the psychological factor is likely the principal key to explain these near-death experiences. Too, one cannot rule out pharmacological, physiological and neurological factors being intertwined with the psychological."

Ryrie goes on to suggest that Satan may be involved in these near-death experiences as well. He says, "A being of light, the identification of which can be adapted to anybody's religious background; a review of one's earthly life with the assurance of forgiveness and acceptance for all; the absence of judgment and eternal punishment: all these factors, so prominent in the researchers' reports, fit perfectly with Satan's clear purpose to counterfeit the truth of God's word."

What are the specific objections that evangelicals and fundamentalists have to accepting the near-death experiences as a revelation from God? Here are a few, which are gathered from Ryrie's writings, Tim LaHaye's *Life in the Afterlife,* and other sources.

• The close brushes with death are often followed by a lessened fear of death. As Scriptural authority to show that being truly in the presence of God would be a fearful rather than soothing thing, evangelicals cite Hebrews 10:31: "It is a fearful thing to fall into the hands of the living God."

Other evangelicals, however, have pointed out a problem with using this verse to attack the validity of the near-death encounters. When taken in context, the argument goes, this statement in the Book of Hebrews is referring to those who are living outside the will of God—those who have sinned deliberately and are facing judgment—but not to those who are living within the will of God. In other words, it may be that the many positive reports we have received about near-death experiences involve people whose lives had been lived in accordance with God's will.

• The near-death experiences provide little if any indication that there is judgment by God for sin. Some evangelicals, in making this point, cite passages like Hebrews 10:27, which refers to "a certain fearful expectation of judgment."

But against this position, other evangelicals have argued that judgment will not come until the end of time (Rev. 20), and so anything that happens today would be prior to that judgment and would not necessarily have to involve anything particularly negative.

• Many of the near-death experiences indicate that God may accept all people, whether they are good or bad, into His eternal presence. Those evangelicals who believe that such an interpretation of the afterlife is invalid cite passages like Matthew 13:40–43, which says that God's angels will separate those who "practice lawlessness" and will throw them into a fiery furnace. But again, as with the issue of God's judgment, others would argue that the near-death experiences occur before judgment and consequently before any separation of good people from bad.

There are many similar arguments that evangelicals can make back and forth about these near-death experiences, but the basic difficulty remains the same: The Bible has nothing definitive to say about the kinds of near-death experiences that we have reported. Also, in the view of many, it seems to have little or nothing to say about what happens immediately after death.

There are some references to what apparently happens just at death, such as the parable of Lazarus and the rich man (Luke 16:19–31), and Jesus' statement to the thief on the cross, "Truly, I say to you, today you will be with me in Paradise" (Luke 23:43). But there is much more that is

161

left unsaid than is said in the Bible about what happens immediately after death.

Our findings, which are somewhat different from those that have come before, would seem to offer no problems to those evangelicals who accept the Bible as spiritually authoritative. As has been mentioned earlier, only a minority of those who had a close brush with death reported a positive experience, and this seems entirely consistent with statements like the one made by Jesus in the Sermon on the Mount: "For the gate is narrow and the way is hard, that leads to life, and those who find it are few." (Matt. 7:14)

Also, since whatever happened to these people with a positive experience occurred before any final judgment, there seems to be no necessary contradiction of the scriptural heaven-hell model. In fact, some of the people we talked to had a sufficiently negative experience to suggest that something like hell may indeed exist.

As for the lessened fear of death in many of those we interviewed, many things could be made of that reaction. It might well be argued by evangelicals that Satan is involved in these experiences and consequently is fooling those who have been near death into thinking that the afterlife will be a positive experience for everyone, no matter what their relationship with God may be.

Evangelicals are first and foremost biblically oriented people, and our near-death accounts are, for the most part, simply not directly covered by scriptural teaching.

As a result, we conclude that our near-death reports are entirely consistent with traditional scriptural interpretations insofar as the Scriptures make suggestions or allusions to things that happened in the near-death encounters. But there are many, many things in the reports we've received that are not covered at all by Scripture. So perhaps evangelical Christians can safely conclude that at least some of our near-death reports may shed extra light on what the afterlife, or at least the afterlife between death and final judgment, is all about.

2. *The Traditional Roman Catholic Viewpoint.* While the evangelical Christian faith is characterized by an emphasis on the individual's literal acceptance of the Bible as true, the traditional Catholic believer looks to the church and its human representative, the pope, as the primary source of spiritual authority. This is not to say that Catholics don't take the Bible very seriously, because they do. But they are not committed to an independent reliance on the Scriptures, as much as on the church's doctrines and interpretations.

The Catholic, like the Protestant, tends to believe, as *The Teaching of Christ* catechism says, ". . . men do not totally die. 'It is appointed for men to die once, and after that comes judgment' (Hebrews 9:27). What we call death is not a complete ceasing to be. Rather, it is a transition to another state of living. 'Lord for your faithful people, life is changed, not ended.' [from Roman Missal, preface I used in Masses for the dead]. One who loves Christ at death does not find death utterly terrible. To die for Christ is 'To depart and to be with Christ' (Phil. 1:23). Nevertheless, death is a great enemy that men naturally fear and hate."

According to their catechism, Catholics also believe that their church members go directly to the presence of God: "They not only enjoy the blessedness of God's immediate presence, the indescribable happiness of knowing and loving God as He knows and loves Himself, but they also contribute to the building of the kingdom by praying for their brothers and sisters in Christ who are still here on earth."

On the other hand, as the catechism indicates, "The dead believer's blessedness is not yet totally fulfilled, for they await the final resurrection and the sharing of that flesh which is part of their being in the joy of eternal life."   163

Roman Catholics also believe in a hell where eternal punishment is levied against those who have consciously rejected God and Christ in this life. Hell consists of eternal separation from God and also sensual pains caused by "the eternal fire" (Matthew 25:41) described in the Scriptures.

As far as we can tell, there have been no official Catholic pronouncements or interpretations of the meaning of some of the near-death accounts. But as with the evangelical position, we can see no particular contradiction between the Catholic outlook on the afterlife and what our studies have revealed.

There are too many uncertainties about the exact vestibule state into which those who have had a close brush with death enter to attempt to compare their experiences with any established church doctrine. Although many of the encounters related to us were quite positive, they may well fall short of the tremendous joy and blessedness expected from God's immediate presence, which Catholics teach is the permanent state of those who have passed away.

3. Liberal Protestants and Catholics. We use the term "liberal" Protestants and Catholics to refer to those who have identified themselves with one of these two religious traditions but who do not take the Bible or the church's teaching as the ultimately definitive spiritual authority.

In other words, those in this category tend to pick and choose those doctrines and scriptural passages that seem valid and true to them personally. But in the last analysis, they tend to rely on their own perceptions about what seems valid in the spiritual realm, including the afterlife.

Because of the highly individualistic nature of the positions held by those in this liberal camp, it's very difficult to generalize about what they believe. As our surveys indicate, a substantial number of people who call themselves Protestants or Catholics do not believe in the existence of the afterlife, heaven or hell.

For example, less than half of all Catholics say they believe in the existence of hell, despite the church's clear teaching that hell does exist. And only about three-quarters of all Protestants and Catholics believe there is definitely a heaven.

Certain liberal theologians like Rudolph Bultmann and Paul Tillich have encouraged this movement toward rejection of biblical authority and traditional doctrine. Tillich, for example, was heard quite often to refer in his lectures at American universities to that "great American superstition, the immortality of the soul."

And as a matter of fact, neither Tillich nor Bultmann devotes much space in his writings to these symbols of heaven and hell. In the index to his classic volume, *Primitive Christianity,* Bultmann has no references to heaven, hell, or immortality—and only three references to death. Tillich, in his three-volume *Systematic Theology,* has a few references to these subjects, but not many in light of the number of pages he gives to other subjects.

If our findings really do reflect some sort of encounters with the supernatural realm, then they do, of course, contradict the views of those like Tillich, Bultmann and other liberal theologians who deny the existence of, or at least anything approximating a traditional view of heaven or hell.

4. Judaism. There is as broad a range of views about the afterlife among contemporary Jews as there is among the various Christian groups. It would be impossible to cover all the variations of Jewish beliefs about the afterlife in one short section in this book. But to get some notion about the spectrum of belief among Jews, it's helpful to begin with the rich historical traditions that gave birth to some of the branches in modern-day Judaism.

In the early books of the Old Testament, little was said about the nature of the afterlife. Generally, the dead seem to have gone to a place called Sheol, but there is almost   165 no indication about what this place may have been like. Apparently the early Jews believed the dead retained their personalities in the afterlife, as can be seen when Samuel returned to chasten King Saul after Saul had used the witch of Endor to summon the prophet forth (1 Samuel 28:7ff). But what their activities were must remain largely to the imagination.

In later books of the Old Testament, the nature of the afterlife became somewhat more clearly defined, with a definite delineation between a place of joy for the good people and of sorrow and pain for the bad.

Gradually, the idea emerged of a sort of hell, called Gehenna. The name comes from the Valley of Ben-Hinnom, which lay just outside the walls of Jerusalem and was once the scene of burning sacrifices of children. The area later became a dump where garbage was burned. Isaiah 66:24 refers to such a place: "And they shall go forth and look on the dead bodies of the men that have rebelled against me; for their worm shall not die, their fire shall not be quenched, and they shall be an abhorrence to all flesh." Later rabbinic writings also identified Gehenna as the pit of fire where evil people are punished after they die.

But these are just some very basic biblical and historical precedents, and from these roots, a wide variety of beliefs about the afterlife have appeared among religious Jews. For example, two religious parties constantly vied with each other for power during the centuries just before and during the early Christian period, and a major point of difference between them was their approach to the afterlife.

One of these groups, the Sadducees, was quite conservative religiously, in that they only accepted the written laws of the Pentateuch, or the five books of the Law in the Old Testament. As a result of this orientation, they are reported to have denied the resurrection of the body after death; the afterlife, including any place of reward or punishment; and the existence of angels and demons.

166

In contrast, their primary opponents, the Pharisees, believed in the immortality of the soul, or as the Roman-Jewish historian Josephus put it: "Every soul, they maintain, is imperishable, but the soul of the good alone passes into another body, while the souls of the wicked suffer eternal punishment."

They also affirmed a resurrection of the body for the blessed after death and a complex set of convictions about a hierarchy of angels in the afterlife.

The Pharisees had a greater long-term historical impact among the Jews than the Sadducees, and their ideas influenced rabbinical thought centuries after they had faded away as an identifiable group. And it's interesting, as we examine Judaism today, that some of the same issues that separated Jewish religious factions more than two millennia ago are still polarizing influences.

Specifically, there are three—and perhaps four—major religious divisions in Judaism today. The main bodies are Orthodox, Conservative, and Reform Judaism, and a growing "reconstructionist" movement makes the fourth. Although many theological and philosophical issues separate these groups and individual sects and congregations within them, their views on the afterlife serve as one of the best barometers of their basic disagreements.

For example, the reconstructionist group tends to be the most liberal in that they stress the "peoplehood" of the Jews but generally discard any notion of the supernatural. In other words, they completely reject the idea that there is any life after death, and so they would be inclined to discount any supernatural interpretation of the near-death experiences we've been presenting in this book.

Reform Jews, whose guiding light was the eighteenth-century Jewish thinker Moses Mendelssohn, have traditionally refused to affirm any point of belief except those which could be ascertained through naked human reason. As a result, the Reform movement has generally rejected the

167

idea of a personal messiah, the supernatural nature of the revelation of God to Moses on Mount Sinai, and any doctrine of resurrection. Reform Jews may, however, affirm a belief in some sort of immortality.

But these religious views change drastically—and, in fact, seem to come closer to some of the convictions of the ancient Pharisees—as we move to the more conservative end of the spectrum of Jewish belief. Conservative and Orthodox Jews often affirm a complex idea of life after death, resurrection of the dead and the eventual appearance of a messiah.

To illustrate, here are a few passages from a *Daily Prayer Book* used in many Conservative synagogues:

• Part of a prayer in the house of mourners: "I believe with perfect faith that there will be a resurrection of the dead at the time when it shall please the Creator, blessed be his name, and exalted be the remembrance of him for ever and ever."

• A selection from "The Memorial of Departed Souls": "May God remember the soul of our honoured father who is gone to his repose; for that, I now solemnly offer charity for his sake; in reward of this, may his soul enjoy eternal life, with the souls of Abraham, Isaac, and Jacob; Sarah, Rebecca, Rachel, and Leah, and the rest of the religious males and females that are in Paradise; and let us say, Amen."

It's clear, from passages like these, that conservative Jews believe that there is a heavenly realm that awaits those who have led good lives on this earth.

Of course, even though certain religious traditions in Judaism or Christianity may appear to offer no obstacle to the possibility that God may be revealing something of Himself in some close brushes with death, there is no necessity to come to this conclusion. As we've already seen, even though a person's religious tradition may encourage such a belief, he may still reject these experiences as a revelation from God on several grounds. He may feel, for example, that they are demon-inspired. Or he may just decide that the arguments of many scientists, who offer physical or psychological explanations, are too convincing to accept a supernatural answer.

But our purpose is not to convince anyone that the reports of those who have been on the verge of death are definitely glimpses of eternity. The views of religious leaders and scientists can only suggest possible directions in which a person can go to seek a final answer. In the last analysis, each individual must sort through his or her own biases, beliefs and basic assumptions about life, and then make the final judgment for himself or herself.

14

The Psychology
of the Afterlife

ALTHOUGH WE'VE MENTIONED elsewhere what
some psychiatrists think about near-death experiences, much still remains to be said about the approach of the sciences of the mind—like psychiatry
and psychology—to this subject.

As a matter of fact, in some ways psychiatrists,
psychologists and those in related disciplines may
be in an even better position than physical scientists
and theologians to evaluate some of these close
brushes with death.

They, more than professionals in any other discipline, are constantly probing the frontiers of unusual
mental activity in their daily work. Also, those in
the mental health field are doing some of the most
creative research to unveil the meaning of the near-
death encounters.

One of the most interesting examples of this type
of work that has come to my attention lately is an
article entitled "Do 'Near Death Experiences' Occur
Only Near Death?" which was published in 1981
in *The Journal of Nervous and Mental Disease* (Vol.
169, No. 6). One of the authors, Dr. Glen O. Gabbard,

is the staff psychiatrist of the Menninger Foundation in Topeka, Kansas.

Gabbard and his colleagues attempted to carry the understanding of out-of-body experiences (or OBEs, as they call them) in near-death experiences (NDEs) one step further. They investigated whether there is anything special about the OBE during a close brush with death, in contrast with the OBE that occurs in other circumstances. In their study of 339 people who reported OBEs, these researchers found "the vast majority of OBEs, 90 percent in our sample, do not occur during a NDE." But was there anything distinctive about that other 10 percent who reported out-of-body experiences *during* a near-death experience?

They concluded that "there are no characteristics which are exclusive to near-death situations." But at the same time, they said, "certain features are impressive inasmuch as they were significantly more often associated with NDEs than with other OBEs." The especially characteristic features of out-of-body sensations that occurred during a verge-of-death incident are that the person is:

• more likely to hear noises during the early stage of the experience;

• more likely to feel he is going through a tunnel;

• more inclined to see his physical body from a distance;

• more apt to sense there are other beings in nonphysical form with him (especially loved ones who have died);

• more likely to encounter a communicative being described as a "brilliant light"; and

• more likely to feel after the near-death incident is over that 1) there is a purpose associated with it, 2) it's an experience of lasting benefit, 3) it's a spiritual or religious experience, and 4) his life is changed by the experience.

As you can see, there are a number of similarities between these findings and the information that our present study has turned up. But it's important to remember the

172

very specific and limited nature of Gabbard's study: He and his associates were concentrating only on the out-of-body experiences that have been reported in near-death incidents. They wanted to see what, if anything, was different or distinctive about the OBEs that occurred in close brushes with death in contrast with those that occurred at other times. Because their objective was narrow and clearly focused, they have succeeded in taking a small but perhaps highly significant step in adding to the total knowledge available about the near-death encounters.

This kind of research, of course, still leaves many unanswered questions. And because certain scientific tools simply aren't available at this point to probe deeper, many physical scientists would probably not be satisfied with the inherent limitations of such work. But as I said before, the very existence of these limitations is one of the reasons that those in the mental health field are in an excellent position to make important contributions.

Another of these mental health experts, who has been given access to our findings and has graciously agreed to offer some comments on them, is Dr. J. William Worden, an assistant professor of psychology at the Harvard Medical School. He holds graduate degrees from Eastern Seminary, Boston University, and Harvard University in the fields of theology, education, and clinical psychology.

For more than a decade Dr. Worden has been the research director of the Omega Project, one of the longest-running studies on life-threatening illness and life-threatening behavior in the country. He is the author of numerous articles and two books, *PDA—Personal Death Awareness* and the recently published *Grief Counseling and Grief Therapy: A Handbook for the Mental Health Practitioner.*

Dr. Worden has had a long-standing interest in near-death experiences, as he indicated to us in this story which he has told in both his writings and his lectures:

"When I was a teenager, our minister announced one 173

Sunday morning that a highly unusual man would speak to us at the church the following Wednesday evening. He was billed as a person who had been medically dead for a brief period and then revived in a hospital. Hearing such a story intrigued me, so I, with several hundred others, crowded into our church basement and waited expectantly for this adventurer who had looked his own death in the face and had lived to tell about it.

"Even now I can recall him—an ordinary-looking man who did not seem the type of person to brave such a perilous encounter. But as he started speaking, I tried to put myself in his shoes and experience what he had been through. I can remember only a few fragments of what he said: 'I had the sense of peace . . . a feeling I was slipping away . . . suspended by some force outside myself . . . perhaps God.'

"It was all very interesting, but much too abbreviated to satisfy me completely. As I left church that evening, I felt a little more hopeful about my own death, a little more informed about what I could expect. But like most others who have heard these accounts of the other side, I wanted to know more. Of course until we die ourselves we can never know exactly what death feels like or what it involves. Still, it's possible to get some immediate sense of the experience if we listen closely to the stories of a number of people who have, in effect, 'died' and come back to life."

As a scholar with a background in both theology and psychology, as well as years of practical experience working with dying patients, Dr. Worden is in a unique position to evaluate some of the information we've discovered. Do these near-death findings reflect some eternal, extradimensional sphere of existence, or are they merely mental movies going on in the brains of those who have responded to our study?

"I would not be in the category of people who believe 174 you can prove these things scientifically," he says. "I take a Pauline point of view, that now we see through a glass darkly, but after death we will know more clearly and fully [from St. Paul's first letter to the Corinthians, chapter 13]. Some may argue that those who believe in life after death are in effect denying death. But you can't prove that position any more than you can prove mine or anyone else's."

His work at the Harvard Medical School has shown him that there are "a lot of biochemical things that go on in learning and in other types of experiences, and you can stimulate different parts of the brain and produce different kinds of perceptual and learning responses. But the problem with the near-death incidents is that no one really knows what is happening on the chemical and molecular level. The natural explanations get as speculative as the religious. You can't subject these experiences to a scientific test—in other words, you can't kill people off and then bring them back. You have to rely on self-reporting, and we know from psychological studies, such as those involving court witnesses who have seen accidents, that biases are built into these accounts. But at the same time, just because there is a limit to our scientific methodology, that doesn't mean that these people haven't had some sort of special experience."

Dr. Worden does raise a number of serious scientific and psychological questions about the near-death reports. Before anyone can get down to the essential, core meaning of any of the close brushes with death, he sees at least four hurdles that must be cleared.

An Epistemological Hurdle. In other words, he explains, "How do we *know* something? How do we evaluate the validity of an individual report of any incident? How much consistency do we need to say that what a given number of people are saying is the same phenomenon, really *is* the same phenomenon? When one of your respondents says

175

he has seen a tunnel, what does that mean exactly? It's hard to get beyond the merely descriptive level because we don't have any externally validating categories of knowledge that allow us to say, with certainty, 'the tunnel perception means this!' "

The High Visibility Hurdle. Sometimes, Dr. Worden says, an individual gets a high visibility or a great sense of importance if he can report an experience that no one else, or only a few other people have had. As a result, there may be a tendency to embroider the experience in the telling, to enhance even further the person's esteem among his fellows.

But there is also another tendency with the near-death type of experience that may act as a corrective on the tendency to exaggerate, according to the Harvard psychologist. He told us, "Sometimes people are quite reluctant to report paranormal phenomena. We had one case involving some bereaved widows who were meeting together in a group to discuss their mutual problems. One of them reported somewhat reluctantly to the group that she had had hallucinations of her dead husband. She quickly found, however, that a number of other women had experienced the same thing—but had decided not to comment on it. The strange experience was normalized by the one woman who had shown the courage to talk about it."

Similarly, we've discovered that a number of people elected not to talk about their near-death encounters, perhaps because they thought others might laugh at them or think them strange. But because of their innate reluctance, it seems that they may be more inclined to be entirely accurate and to avoid exaggeration.

The Popular Mind-set Hurdle. Because there has been a great deal written about near-death encounters in recent years, there may be a tendency for some people to report

176

their sensations in terms of what they have read, rather than what they have actually experienced.

"There are all kinds of problems in getting a handle on this," Dr. Worden says. "If you can't quite find the words to express what happened to you, it's easy to fall back on your newspaper reading or your personal religious background for terminology." As a result, it's sometimes hard to distinguish between the content of the person's near-death encounter and the content of his previous reading and life experiences.

The Trauma Hurdle. "It seems that all of your findings stem from some traumatic incident, such as an accident or a serious operation. There aren't any people who are dying or have come near death from a long illness, like cancer. We know that when physical trauma occurs, important chemical reactions and other changes may occur in the body. Things like endorphins, which help reduce pain, may be released in the brain. When a trauma occurs to the body, you assume a lot of juices flow. We also know that the chemical interplays in the brain may trigger neuro-transmitting agencies, or neurons that transmit information of one sort or another. What effect may this sort of thing have on the near-death reports you've received? At this point, it's hard to say. But this is a scientific hurdle which must be cleared before we can move toward a definitive evaluation of the meaning of the near-death incidents."

So Dr. Worden has pointed up some areas where research must be directed in the future if we hope to come closer to the real meaning of the near-death encounters. But he also has one word of caution for all our readers, which I think it's important to emphasize at this time: "One problem that has bothered me in my research on life-threatening situations is the actions that certain information may prompt people in a depressed state to take.

"Some might read about reincarnation, for example, and begin to believe in it. They might think that there is a better way of life that awaits them their next time around on this earth, and they could decide to opt out of this life altogether. In other words, if you could prove to them that reincarnation actually occurs, they might commit suicide to escape to what they perceive as something better. That's a phenomenon I've seen happen a few times. There are not huge numbers of people who would take their own lives for this reason, but there are some. So it's a danger which we should point out and try to guard against as we discuss these issues relating to the afterlife."

What is Dr. Worden's view on the near-death experience as an intimation of immortality?

"I relegate it to the realm of mystery," he concludes. "My final word would be to say, let's be surprised! You could hold a strong belief that these incidents reflect a life after death, but you could not hold that belief from an epistemological source, or source of knowledge, that is rooted in science. Your source of knowledge, at this point in time, would have to be something else, such as Scripture and divine revelation."

It's clear from these scientific, religious and psychological evaluations that there is disagreement about exactly what these near-death accounts mean.

They may be simply dramatic internal scenarios that are played out entirely in the minds of those who undergo physical traumas. Many scientists and physicians would agree with this interpretation.

Or they may be part of a demonic strategy to trick human beings into thinking the afterlife and the requirements for salvation are different from certain theological positions. Some religious thinkers would explain them this way.

Or might any of the near-death reports be about an actual encounter with the first stages of heaven, or a multidimensional, parallel universe? There are also those who would respond in the affirmative here.

178

Whatever these experiences represent—a physical metamorphosis brought on by the approach of death or a spiritual window providing an actual look beyond the threshold of death—the mere fact of their occurrence may tell us something about our own human nature. They hold a fascination for us that transcends a question of belief or proof.

Personally, I prefer to keep an open mind as to what the near-death reports may really mean. There are certainly strong scientific and theological arguments stating that the near-death adventures may have nothing to do with the afterlife or heaven. But at the same time, the scientific explanations fall short of being completely convincing because at this stage they rest more on speculation than on hard facts or evidence. So it seems best at least to remain open to the possibility that many of those who have had a "strange encounter" during their close brush with death *may* have had some sort of adventure in immortality.

Or to use the words of psychologist J. William Worden, I suppose you might say that I'm ready to be "surprised" at whatever the future may bring forth.

Appendix

LIFE AFTER DEATH?

The question: *Do you believe in life after death, or not?*

	YES	NO	NO OPINION
	%	%	%
NATIONAL	67	27	6
Sex			
Male	61	30	9
Female	72	24	4
Race			
White	69	25	6
Nonwhite	54	38	8
Education			
College	69	25	6
High school	67	27	6
Grade school	62	30	8
Region			
East	56	34	10
Midwest	73	21	6
South	75	22	3
West	61	32	7
Age			
Total under 30	68	26	6
18–24 years	67	26	7
25–29 years	69	25	6
30–49 years	67	27	6
50 & older	67	26	7
Income			
$25,000 & over	66	29	5
$20,000–$24,999	70	22	8
$15,000–$19,999	67	26	7
$10,000–$14,999	72	24	4
$5,000–$9,999	62	29	9
Under $5,000	61	30	9

The question: *Do you believe in life after death, or not?*
(continued)

	YES	NO	NO OPINION
	%	%	%
Protestant Denomination			
Baptist	71	24	5
Methodist	79	18	3
Lutheran	79	12	9
Religion			
Protestant	74	22	4
Catholic	64	28	8
Occupation			
Professional & business	67	26	7
Clerical & sales	62	34	4
Manual workers	68	26	6
Nonlabor force	69	26	5
City Size			
1,000,000 & over	55	36	9
500,000–999,999	62	29	9
50,000–499,999	66	29	5
2,500–49,999	74	22	4
Under 2,500, rural	74	20	6

The question: *In what ways do you think life after death will be different from your present life? Please be as specific as you can about what you believe.*

	NATIONAL
No more problems/troubles	26%
Better/good life	21
Peaceful	16
No sickness/pain	15
Happy/joyful/no sorrow	15

Note Survey results for Jews, members of Eastern Orthodox churches, Presbyterians, Episcopalians, and other denominations are not reported, due to the relatively small sample base for each of these groups.

The question: *In what ways do you think life after death will be different from your present life? Please be as specific as you can about what you believe.* (continued)

	NATIONAL
Spiritual/not physical	13
Be with God/Jesus	8
Perfect/complete	6
Totally different	6
Be in Heaven	4
Love	4
Soul without body	4
Reunion of friends/relatives	3
Eternal	3
Beautiful/glorious	3
Either Heaven or Hell	3
A new body	2
No husbands/wives	*
Miscellaneous	7
Don't know	12
	171%**

* Less than 1%.

** Total adds to more than 67% (the proportion who believe in an afterlife) due to multiple responses.

IS THERE A HELL?

The question: *Do you think there is a Hell, to which people who had led bad lives without being sorry are eternally damned?*

	YES	NO	DON'T KNOW
	%	%	%
NATIONAL	53	37	10
Sex			
Male	50	37	13
Female	55	38	7
Race			
White	53	38	9
Nonwhite	55	33	12

185

The question: *Do you think there is a Hell, to which people who had led bad lives without being sorry are eternally damned?* (continued)

	YES	NO	DON'T KNOW
	%	%	%
Education			
College	47	46	7
High school	54	35	11
Grade school	63	27	10
Region			
East	41	46	13
Midwest	57	34	9
South	72	22	6
West	36	53	11
Age			
Total under 30	53	36	11
18–24 years	56	32	12
25–29 years	47	43	10
30–49 years	53	37	10
50 & older	53	38	9
Income			
$25,000 & over	47	43	10
$20,000–$24,999	58	37	5
$15,000–$19,999	56	34	10
$10,000–$14,999	53	38	9
$5,000–$9,999	54	34	12
Under $5,000	61	31	8
Protestant Denomination			
Baptist	73	19	8
Methodist	56	35	9
Lutheran	63	31	6
Religion			
Protestant	61	30	9
Catholic	48	40	12
Occupation			
Professional & business	46	43	11
Clerical & sales	45	48	7
Manual workers	56	34	10
Nonlabor force	54	37	9

The question: *Do you think there is a Hell, to which people who had led bad lives without being sorry are eternally damned?* (continued)

	YES	NO	DON'T KNOW
	%	%	%
City Size			
1,000,000 & over	41	45	14
500,000–999,999	42	48	10
50,000–499,999	53	39	8
2,500–49,999	58	34	8
Under 2,500, rural	64	27	9

IS THERE A HEAVEN?

The question: *Do you think there is a Heaven where people who had led good lives are eternally rewarded?*

	YES	NO	DON'T KNOW
	%	%	%
NATIONAL	71	21	8
Sex			
Male	66	24	10
Female	75	20	5
Race			
White	71	22	7
Nonwhite	69	19	12
Education			
College	60	33	7
High school	75	17	8
Grade school	77	15	8
Region			
East	61	30	9
Midwest	76	17	7
South	84	11	5
West	58	33	9

The question: *Do you think there is a Heaven where people who have led good lives are eternally rewarded?* (continued)

	YES	NO	DON'T KNOW
	%	%	%
Age			
Total under 30	72	20	8
18–24 years	75	17	8
25–29 years	67	25	8
30–49	70	22	8
50 & older	70	22	8
Income			
$25,000 & over	63	30	7
$20,000–$24,999	71	26	3
$15,000–$19,999	76	16	8
$10,000–$14,999	73	20	7
$5,000–$9,999	75	18	7
Under $5,000	75	13	12
Protestant Denomination			
Baptist	81	12	7
Methodist	81	16	3
Lutheran	78	17	5
Religion			
Protestant	77	17	6
Catholic	73	17	10
Occupation			
Professional & business	61	31	8
Clerical & sales	63	31	6
Manual workers	75	18	7
Nonlabor force	75	17	8
City Size			
1,000,000 & over	58	29	13
500,000–999,999	61	32	7
50,000–499,999	72	21	7
2,500–49,999	77	19	4
Under 2,500, rural	80	13	7

CHANCES OF GOING TO HEAVEN

The question: *Here is an interesting question. . . . How would you describe your own chances of going to Heaven—excellent, good, only fair, or poor?*
(Based on those who think there is a Heaven)

	EXCEL-LENT	GOOD	ONLY FAIR	POOR	NO OPINION
	%	%	%	%	%
NATIONAL	20	44	29	4	3
Sex					
Male	17	40	33	7	3
Female	23	47	26	2	2
Race					
White	20	45	28	4	3
Nonwhite	21	39	35	3	2
Education					
College	24	51	22	1	2
High school	17	42	33	5	3
Grade school	24	39	28	5	4
Region					
East	16	47	32	3	2
Midwest	24	45	26	3	2
South	21	41	29	6	3
West	16	43	32	3	6
Age					
Total under 30	17	42	36	3	2
18–24 years	16	44	34	3	3
25–29 years	20	37	38	4	1
30–49 years	20	43	28	6	3
50 & older	22	46	26	3	3
Income					
$25,000 & over	15	48	30	3	4
$20,000–$24,999	19	44	28	6	3
$15,000–$19,999	21	41	33	4	1
$10,000–$14,999	19	44	28	7	2
$5,000–$9,999	25	42	29	3	1
Under $5,000	21	40	31	4	4

189

The question: *Here is an interesting question. . . . How would you describe your own chances of going to Heaven—excellent, good, only fair, or poor?* (Based on those who think there is a Heaven)

(continued)

	EXCEL-LENT	GOOD	ONLY FAIR	POOR	NO OPINION
	%	%	%	%	%
Protestant Denomination					
Baptist	26	39	27	5	3
Methodist	16	51	28	5	*
Lutheran	20	51	29	*	*
Religion					
Protestant	24	42	28	4	2
Catholic	41	49	31	3	3
Occupation					
Professional & business	23	49	23	2	3
Clerical & sales	28	41	25	4	2
Manual workers	14	41	36	6	3
Nonlabor force	26	45	25	2	2
City					
1,000,000 & over	19	50	26	1	4
500,000–999,999	17	51	28	3	1
50,000–499,999	21	39	34	4	2
2,500–49,999	19	41	32	6	2
Under 2,500, rural	21	44	26	5	4

* Less than 1%.

The question: *Please read this carefully and tell me which of these words or terms apply to your beliefs about life after death or heaven?* (Based on total sample)

	NATIONAL
It will be peaceful	65%
One will be in the presence of God or Jesus Christ	54
God's love will be the center of life after death	54

The question: *Please read this carefully and tell me which of these words or terms apply to your beliefs about life after death or heaven?*

(continued)

	NATIONAL
There will be love between people	53%
One will be happy	52
One will see friends, relatives, spouses	42
One will live forever	42
Crippled people will be whole	38
One will grow spiritually	36
There will be humor	25
There will be angels or devils	23
One will be recognizable as the same person as on earth	21
People will minister to the spiritual needs of others	20
People will have responsibilities	19
One will grow intellectually	18
People will have human form	14
There will be some sort of contact with people on earth	12
People will be the same age as when they die	11
One will be able to minister to the spiritual needs of people on earth	10
One will enjoy material comforts	8
Boring	5
There will be total darkness	5
None of these	13
No answer	3

BELIEVE IN REINCARNATION?

The question: *Do you believe in reincarnation—that is, the rebirth of the soul in a new body after death—or not?*

	YES	NO	NO OPINION
	%	%	%
National	23	67	10
Sex			
Male	21	70	9
Female	25	65	10
Race			
White	23	68	9
Nonwhite	25	62	13
Education			
College	20	71	9
High school	26	66	8
Grade school	22	63	15
Region			
East	23	67	10
Midwest	22	71	7
South	22	68	10
West	27	63	10
Age			
Total under 30	29	61	10
18–24 years	30	61	9
25–29 years	29	61	10
30–49 years	21	68	11
50 & older	21	71	8
Income			
$25,000 & over	22	70	8
$20,000–$24,999	21	70	9
$15,000–$19,999	24	66	10
$10,000–$14,999	22	70	8
$5,000–$9,999	23	64	13
Under $5,000	29	62	9

The question: *Do you believe in reincarnation—that is, the rebirth of the soul in a new body after death—or not?* (continued)

	YES	NO	NO OPINION
	%	%	%
Protestant Denomination			
Baptist	21	70	9
Methodist	26	61	13
Lutheran	22	68	10
Religion			
Protestant	21	68	11
Catholic	25	68	7
Occupation			
Professional & business	23	66	11
Clerical & sales	27	64	9
Manual workers	25	66	9
Nonlabor force	20	72	8
City Size			
1,000,000 & over	26	65	9
500,000–999,999	25	61	14
50,000–499,999	27	66	7
2,500–49,999	19	71	10
Under 2,500, rural	19	71	10

HUMAN LIFE ON OTHER PLANETS?

The question: *Do you believe there is human life on other planets, or not?*

	YES	NO	NO OPINION
	%	%	%
NATIONAL	46	41	13
Sex			
Male	50	37	13
Female	43	44	13
Race			
White	47	41	12
Nonwhite	35	43	22

The question: *Do you believe there is human life on other planets, or not?* (continued)

	YES	NO	NO OPINION
	%	%	%
Education			
College	45	43	12
High school	49	39	12
Grade school	36	47	17
Region			
East	50	36	14
Midwest	45	40	15
South	37	48	15
West	54	39	7
Age			
Total under 30	55	35	10
18–24 years	54	36	10
25–29 years	57	31	12
30–49 years	47	40	13
50 & older	38	47	15
Income			
$25,000 & over	53	38	9
$20,000–$24,999	45	45	10
$15,000–$19,999	46	40	14
$10,000–$14,999	43	42	15
$5,000–$9,999	44	41	15
Under $5,000	34	47	19
Protestant Denomination			
Baptist	36	48	16
Methodist	55	32	13
Lutheran	39	48	13
Religion			
Protestant	43	43	14
Catholic	52	37	11
Occupation			
Professional & business	49	40	11
Clerical & sales	50	41	9
Manual workers	49	39	12
Nonlabor force	37	47	16

194

The question: *Do you believe there is human life on other planets, or not?*

	YES	NO	NO OPINION
	%	%	%
City Size			
1,000,000 & over	43	43	14
500,000–999,999	52	38	10
50,000–499,999	47	43	10
2,500–49,999	45	42	13
Under 2,500, rural	45	39	16

CONTACT WITH THE DEAD?

The question: *Do you think it is possible to have contact with the dead, or not?*

	YES	NO	NO OPINION
	%	%	%
NATIONAL	24	69	7
Sex			
Male	21	70	9
Female	26	69	5
Race			
White	24	69	7
Nonwhite	18	69	13
Education			
College	28	66	6
High school	25	67	8
Grade school	9	83	8
Region			
East	25	67	8
Midwest	22	70	8
South	18	75	7
West	33	61	6
Age			
Total under 30	38	54	8
18–24 years	36	56	8
25–29 years	43	50	7
30–49 years	24	68	8
50 & older	12	82	6

195

The question: *Do you think it is possible to have contact with the dead, or not?* (continued)

	YES	NO	NO OPINION
	%	%	%
Income			
$25,000 & over	25	69	6
$20,000–24,999	25	69	6
$15,000–$19,999	27	65	8
$10,000–$14,999	27	67	6
$5,000–$9,999	17	73	10
Under $5,000	19	73	8
Protestant Denomination			
Baptist	15	80	5
Methodist	25	63	12
Lutheran	23	75	2
Religion			
Protestant	20	73	7
Catholic	26	65	9
Occupation			
Professional & business	26	68	6
Clerical & sales	28	63	9
Manual workers	27	65	8
Nonlabor force	16	80	4
City Size			
1,000,000 & over	28	64	8
500,000–999,999	34	59	7
50,000–499,999	25	70	5
2,500–49,999	20	70	10
Under 2,500, rural	16	76	8

WILL LIFE AFTER DEATH
BE SCIENTIFICALLY PROVED?

The question: *Do you think life after death will ever be proved scientifically, or not?*

	YES	NO	NO OPINION
	%	%	%
NATIONAL	20	68	12
Sex			
Male	17	71	12
Female	24	64	12
Race			
White	21	68	11
Nonwhite	20	62	18
Education			
College	21	70	9
High school	22	67	11
Grade school	14	66	20
Region			
East	22	64	14
Midwest	18	68	14
South	18	71	11
West	25	68	7
Age			
Total under 30	29	62	9
18–24 years	30	62	8
25–29 years	27	63	10
30–49 years	17	69	14
50 & older	18	70	12
Income			
$25,000 & over	23	67	10
$20,000–$24,999	19	74	7
$15,000–$19,999	20	68	12
$10,000–$14,999	18	70	12
$5,000–$9,999	20	63	17
Under $5,000	21	66	13

The question: *Do you think life after death will ever be proved scientifically, or not?* (continued)

	YES	NO	NO OPINION
Protestant Denomination			
Baptist	17	70	13
Methodist	24	63	13
Lutheran	15	74	11
Religion			
Protestant	20	68	12
Catholic	21	68	11
Occupation			
Professional & business	21	70	9
Clerical & sales	25	60	15
Manual workers	23	66	11
Nonlabor force	15	71	14
City Size			
1,000,000 & over	24	63	13
500,000–999,999	23	67	10
50,000–499,999	19	69	12
2,500–49,999	22	68	10
Under 2,500, rural	18	69	13

VERGE-OF-DEATH EXPERIENCES?

The question: *Here is a question about unusual experiences people say they have had when they have been on the verge of death or have had a "close call" such as experiences of continued life or an awareness after death. Have you, yourself, ever been on the verge of death or had a "close call" which involved any unusual experience at that time?*

	YES	NO	NOT SURE
	%	%	%
NATIONAL	15	83	2
Sex			
Male	17	82	1
Female	13	84	3

198

The question: *Here is a question about unusual experiences people say they have had when they have been on the verge of death or have had a "close call" such as experiences of continued life or an awareness after death. Have you, yourself, ever been on the verge of death or had a "close call" which involved any unusual experience at that time?* (continued)

	YES %	NO %	NOT SURE %
Race			
White	15	84	1
Nonwhite	17	75	8
Education			
College	13	86	1
High school	15	83	2
Grade school	19	77	4
Region			
East	16	82	2
Midwest	12	86	2
South	13	84	3
West	20	79	1
Age			
Total under 30	11	88	1
18–24 years	10	89	1
25–29 years	13	86	1
30–49 years	15	81	3
50 & older	17	81	2
Income			
$25,000 & over	14	85	1
$20,000–$24,999	12	87	1
$15,000–$19,999	14	84	2
$10,000–$14,999	15	82	3
$5,000–$9,999	18	79	3
Under $5,000	19	77	4
Protestant Denomination			
Baptist	14	83	3
Methodist	17	81	2
Lutheran	13	85	2

199

The question: *Here is a question about unusual ex-periences people say they have had when they have been on the verge of death or have had a "close call" such as experiences of continued life or an awareness after death. Have you, yourself, ever been on the verge of death or had a "close call" which involved any unusual experience at that time?* (continued)

	YES	NO	NOT SURE
	%	%	%
Religion			
Protestant	16	82	2
Catholic	13	86	1
Occupation			
Professional & business	14	85	1
Clerical & sales	13	83	4
Manual workers	15	83	2
Nonlabor force	19	79	2
City Size			
1,000,000 & over	15	83	2
500,000–999,999	20	78	2
50,000–499,999	12	86	2
2,500–49,999	14	85	1
Under 2,500, rural	16	82	2

DESCRIPTION OF VERGE-OF-DEATH EXPERIENCE

(Based on the 15 percent who had an experience)

An overwhelming sense of peace and painlessness	11%
A fast review or reexamination of the individual's life	11
A special sensation of feeling, such as the impression of being in an entirely different world	11
The out-of-body sensation	9

200

An acute visual perception of surroundings and events during the near-death experience	8
A feeling that a special being or beings were present during the near-death experience	8
The presence of a blindingly bright light or series of lights	5
Perception of a tunnel	3
Premonitions of some future event or events	2
A sense of hell, torment	1
Description of serious illness, accidents, etc.	60
Other responses	2
No opinion	4
	135*

* Total adds to more than 100 percent due to multiple responses.

The following figures reflect the nationwide responses to some of the major questions in our surveys in terms of personal religious involvement. The tables should be read *down* to ascertain the proper responses. For example, in the first set of figures, read as follows: "Among those involved in regular attendance at a church or synagogue, 77 percent responded, 'yes,' they believe in life after death."

	CHURCH ATTENDANCE	
	YES	NO
Life After Death?		
Yes	77%	61%
No	18	32
No opinion	5	7
Is There a Hell?		
Yes	66	45
No	26	44
Don't know	8	11
Is There a Heaven?		
Yes	85	62
No	11	28
Don't know	4	10

201

	CHURCH ATTENDANCE	
	YES	NO
Believe in Reincarnation?		
Yes	17%	27%
No	74	63
No opinion	9	10
Human Life on Other Planets?		
Yes	37	52
No	47	37
No opinion	16	11
Contact the Dead?		
Yes	18	27
No	74	66
No opinion	8	7
Life After Death Scientifically Proved?		
Yes	17	23
No	71	65
No opinion	12	12
Verge-of-Death Experience?		
Yes	13	16
No	84	82
Not sure	3	2

	CHURCH MEMBERSHIP	
	YES	NO
Life After Death?		
Yes	74%	53%
No	21	38
No opinion	5	9
Is There a Hell?		
Yes	60	38
No	32	49
Don't know	8	13

	CHURCH MEMBERSHIP	
	YES	NO
Is There a Heaven?		
Yes	79	55
No	16	33
Don't know	5	12
Believe in Reincarnation?		
Yes	21	28
No	70	61
No opinion	9	11
Human Life on Other Planets?		
Yes	43	52
No	43	37
No opinion	14	11
Contact the Dead?		
Yes	21	28
No	72	63
No opinion	7	9
Life After Death Scientifically Proved?		
Yes	20	22
No	68	66
No opinion	12	12
Verge-of-Death Experience?		
Yes	15	16
No	83	83
Not sure	2	1

	IMPORTANCE OF RELIGION IN LIFE		
	VERY	FAIRLY	NOT VERY
Life After Death?			
Yes	80%	60%	39%
No	16	33	51
No opinion	4	7	10
Is There a Hell?			
Yes	68	44	19
No	25	44	66
Don't know	7	12	15

	IMPORTANCE OF RELIGION IN LIFE		
	VERY	FAIRLY	NOT VERY
Is There a Heaven?			
Yes	87%	64%	29%
No	9	26	58
Don't know	4	10	13
Believe in Reincarnation?			
Yes	22	25	27
No	70	65	63
No opinion	8	10	10
Human Life on Other Planets?			
Yes	40	52	56
No	43	41	34
No opinion	17	7	10
Contact the Dead?			
Yes	21	26	27
No	72	66	66
No opinion	7	8	7
Life After Death Scientifically Proved?			
Yes	19	21	24
No	69	68	65
No opinion	12	11	11
Verge-of-Death Experience?			
Yes	17	12	14
No	81	86	84
Not sure	2	2	2

	HAD RELIGIOUS EXPERIENCE	
	YES	NO
Life After Death?		
Yes	83%	60%
No	12	33
No opinion	5	7

	HAD RELIGIOUS EXPERIENCE	
	YES	NO
Is There a Hell?		
Yes	72%	44%
No	22	45
Don't know	6	11
Is There a Heaven?		
Yes	86	64
No	11	27
Don't know	3	9
Believe in Reincarnation?		
Yes	25	22
No	66	69
No opinion	9	9
Human Life on Other Planets?		
Yes	43	48
No	41	41
No opinion	16	11
Contact the Dead?		
Yes	29	21
No	64	72
No opinion	7	7
Life After Death Scientifically Proved?		
Yes	21	20
No	68	68
No opinion	11	12
Verge-of-Death Experience?		
Yes	23	11
No	75	87
Not sure	2	2

	HAD RELIGIOUS EXPERIENCE THAT INVOLVED CHRIST	
	YES	NO
Life After Death?		
Yes	85%	67%
No	11	19
No opinion	4	14
Is There a Hell?		
Yes	77	25
No	17	65
Don't know	6	10
Is There a Heaven?		
Yes	90	49
No	7	47
Don't know	3	4
Believe in Reincarnation?		
Yes	23	43
No	69	38
No opinion	8	19
Human Life on Other Planets?		
Yes	41	54
No	42	35
No opinion	17	10
Contact the Dead?		
Yes	26	49
No	67	45
No opinion	7	6
Life After Death Scientifically Proved?		
Yes	20	34
No	69	52
No opinion	11	14
Verge-of-Death Experience?		
Yes	21	41
No	77	55
Not sure	2	4

1981 SURVEY ON BELIEFS OF LEADING
SCIENTISTS ABOUT LIFE AFTER DEATH

LIFE AFTER DEATH?

Do you believe in life after death, or not?

Yes	16%
No	68
No opinion	16
	100%

IS THERE A HELL?

Do you think there is a Hell, to which people who have led bad lives and die without being sorry are eternally damned?

Yes	4%
No	80
No opinion	16
	100%

IS THERE A HEAVEN?

Do you think there is a heaven, where people who have led good lives are eternally rewarded?

Yes	8%
No	76
No opinion	16
	100%

PEOPLE MINISTER TO NEEDS OF OTHERS?

If you believe in life after death, do you think people in the afterlife will minister to the needs of others?

Yes	4%
No	7
No opinion	40
Don't believe	49
	100%

CHANCES OF GOING TO HEAVEN?

How would you describe YOUR OWN chances of going to heaven—excellent, good, only fair, or poor?

Excellent	7%
Good	5
Only fair	4
Poor	0
No opinion	15
Don't believe	69
	100%

BELIEVE IN REINCARNATION?

Do you believe in reincarnation—that is, rebirth of the soul in a new body after death, or not?

Yes	8
No	77
No opinion	15
	100%

HUMAN LIFE ON OTHER PLANETS?

Do you believe there is human life on other planets, or not?

Yes	35%
No	33
No opinion	32

POSSIBLE TO HAVE CONTACT WITH THE DEAD?

Do you think it is possible to have contact with the dead, or not?

Yes	5%
No	82
No opinion	13
	100%

WILL LIFE AFTER DEATH BE SCIENTIFICALLY PROVED?

Do you think life after death will ever be proved scientifically or not?

Yes	4%
No	74
No opinion	22
	100%

EVER HAD SUPERNATURAL EXPERIENCE?

Have you ever had what you regard as an encounter with an angel or a devil, or some other kind of supernatural experience?

Yes	5%
No	85
No opinion	10
	100%

VERGE-OF-DEATH EXPERIENCE?

Here is a question about unusual experiences people say they have had when they had been on the verge of death or have had a "close call"—such as experiences of continued life or an awareness after death. Have you, yourself, ever been on the verge of death or had a close call which involved any unusual experience at that time?

Yes	10%
No	81
Not sure	3
No opinion	6
	100%

Note   The above results are based on a small but representative sample of persons in the field of science, drawn at random from Marquis's *Who's Who in America.*

1981 SURVEY ON BELIEFS OF LEADING SCIENTISTS ABOUT LIFE AFTER DEATH

LIFE AFTER DEATH?

Do you believe in life after death, or not?

Yes	32%
No	60
No opinion	8
	100%

IS THERE A HELL?

Do you think there is a Hell, to which people who have led bad lives and die without being sorry are eternally damned?

Yes	15%
No	73
No opinion	12
	100%

IS THERE A HEAVEN?

Do you think there is a heaven, where people who have led good lives are eternally rewarded?

Yes	24%
No	67
No opinion	9
	100%

PEOPLE MINISTER TO NEEDS OF OTHERS?

If you believe in life after death, do you think people in the afterlife will minister to the needs of others?

Yes	8%
No	16
No opinion	36
Don't believe	40
	100%

CHANCES OF GOING TO HEAVEN?

How would you describe your own *chances of going to heaven—excellent, good, only fair, or poor?*

Excellent	9%
Good	15
Only fair	5
Poor	0
No opinion	14
Don't believe	57
	100%

BELIEVE IN REINCARNATION?

Do you believe in reincarnation—that is, rebirth of the soul in a new body after death, or not?

Yes	9%
No	82
No opinion	9
	100%

HUMAN LIFE ON OTHER PLANETS?
Do you believe there is human life on other planets, or not?

Yes	25%
No	39
No opinion	36
	100%

POSSIBLE TO HAVE CONTACT WITH THE DEAD?
Do you think it is possible to have contact with the dead, or not?

Yes	9%
No	78
No opinion	13
	100%

WILL LIFE AFTER DEATH BE SCIENTIFICALLY PROVED?
Do you think life after death will ever be proved scientifically or not?

Yes	5%
No	75
No opinion	20
	100%

EVER HAD SUPERNATURAL EXPERIENCE?
Have you ever had what you regard as an encounter with an angel or a devil, or some other kind of supernatural experience?

Yes	3%
No	86
No opinion	11
	100%

VERGE-OF-DEATH EXPERIENCE?

Here is a question about unusual experiences people say they have had when they had been on the verge of death or have had a "close call"—such as experiences of continued life or an awareness after death. Have you, yourself, ever been on the verge of death or had a close call which involved any unusual experience at that time?

Yes	9%
No	86
Not sure	1
No opinion	4
	100%

Note The above results are based on a small but representative sample of persons in the field of medicine, drawn at random from Marquis's *Who's Who in America.*

The question: *Do you think your soul will live on after death?*

	1965			1952		
	YES	NO	DON'T KNOW	YES	NO	DON'T KNOW
	%	%	%	%	%	%
TOTAL	75	10	15	77	7	16
Religion						
Roman Catholic	83	3	14	85	4	11
Protestant total	78	7	15	80	5	15
Baptist	81	5	14	87	2	11
Methodist	75	7	18	77	6	17
Lutheran	78	7	15	78	6	16
Presbyterian	70	11	19	80	7	13
Episcopal	68	15	17	67	7	26
Congregational	65	11	24	63	15	22
Other denominations	83	8	9	78	7	15
Jewish	17	46	37	35	24	41
Other and none	37	42	21	43	25	32
Sex						
Men	72	13	15	75	8	17
Women	77	7	16	80	5	15

The question: *Do you think your soul will live on after death?*

	1965			1952		
	YES	NO	DON'T KNOW	YES	NO	DON'T KNOW
	%	%	%	%	%	%
Age						
18–24 years	73	13	14	75	7	18
25–34	74	11	15	76	7	17
35–44	73	9	18	77	7	16
45–54	73	10	17	76	7	17
55–64	76	9	15	80	6	14
65 & over	79	8	13	81	5	14
Race						
White	76	9	15	77	7	16
Nonwhite	61	16	23	79	4	17
Education						
0–8th grade	78	6	16	76	7	17
1–3 years high school	74	9	17	75	6	19
High school graduate	75	10	15	81	4	15
1–3 years college	77	12	11	78	7	15
College graduate	66	15	19	72	16	12
Occupation						
Professional	73	12	15	77	10	13
Proprietor or manager	77	10	13	74	9	17
White-collar worker	73	9	18	83	4	13
Service worker	72	12	16	80	7	13
Manual worker	75	9	16	76	6	18
Farmer	84	4	12	83	3	14
Nonlabor force	74	10	16	–	–	–
Income						
Upper	73	13	14	77	7	16
Middle	74	11	15	79	6	15
Lower	76	7	17	76	7	17
City Size						
Over 1 Million	65	16	19	70	10	20
100,000–1 Million	71	11	18	75	8	17
25,000–100,000	83	4	13	76	7	17
10,000–25,000	76	11	13	72	6	22
Under 10,000	81	6	13	81	6	13
Rural, farm	84	4	12	82	3	15
Region						
New England	67	17	16	78	7	15
Middle Atlantic	69	13	18	72	8	20
South Atlantic	80	5	15	82	4	14
East South Central	93	2	5	87	3	10

The question: *Do you think your soul will live on after death?*
(continued)

	1965			1952		
	YES	NO	DON'T KNOW	YES	NO	DON'T KNOW
	%	%	%	%	%	%
West South Central	80	5	15	87	3	10
East North Central	75	9	16	74	8	18
West North Central	80	8	12	79	3	18
Mountain	75	14	11	72	11	17
Pacific	65	15	20	76	9	15

The question: *Do you think there is a Heaven, where people who have led good lives are eternally rewarded?*

	1965				1952			
	BELIEVE IN AFTERLIFE			DON'T BELIEVE IN AFTERLIFE	BELIEVE IN AFTERLIFE			DON'T BELIEVE IN AFTERLIFE
	YES	NO	DON'T KNOW		YES	NO	DON'T KNOW	
	%	%	%	%	%	%	%	%
TOTAL	68	3	4	25	72	2	3	23
Religion								
Roman Catholic	80	1	2	17	83	1	1	15
Protestant total	71	3	4	22	75	2	3	20
Baptist	78	1	2	19	83	1	3	13
Methodist	66	3	6	25	72	1	4	23
Lutheran	66	3	9	22	74	2	2	22
Presbyterian	61	3	7	29	71	3	6	20
Episcopal	54	10	4	32	58	4	5	33
Congregational	58	4	3	35	59	4	*	37
Other denominations	75	3	5	17	71	4	3	22
Jewish	6	5	6	83	21	5	9	65
Other and none	26	7	4	63	40	1	2	57
Sex								
Men	65	3	4	28	70	2	3	25
Women	70	3	4	23	75	2	3	20
Age								
18–24 years	68	3	2	27	70	3	2	25
25–34	66	4	4	26	71	2	3	24
35–44	67	2	4	27	72	2	3	23
45–54	67	2	4	27	71	2	3	24
55–64	71	2	3	24	74	2	4	20
65 & over	70	3	6	21	76	2	3	19

The question: *Do you think there is a Heaven, where people who have led good lives are eternally rewarded?*

(continued)

	1965				1952			
	BELIEVE IN AFTERLIFE			DON'T BELIEVE IN AFTERLIFE	BELIEVE IN AFTERLIFE			DON'T BELIEVE IN AFTERLIFE
	YES	NO	DON'T KNOW		YES	NO	DON'T KNOW	
	%	%	%	%	%	%	%	%
Race								
White	69	3	4	24	72	2	3	23
Nonwhite	57	3	1	39	72	3	4	21
Education								
0–8th grade	74	1	3	22	73	1	2	24
1–3 years high school	72	1	1	26	70	1	4	25
High school graduate	68	3	4	25	77	2	2	19
1–3 years college	67	4	6	23	69	5	4	22
College graduate	51	6	9	34	60	5	7	28
Occupation								
Professional	61	7	5	27	68	4	5	23
Proprietor or manager	68	3	6	23	68	2	4	26
White-collar worker	65	4	4	27	76	3	4	17
Service worker	68	1	3	28	75	2	3	20
Manual worker	70	2	3	25	72	1	3	24
Farmer	82	1	1	16	81	*	2	17
Nonlabor force	66	2	6	26	*	*	*	*
Income								
Upper	62	5	6	27	70	3	4	23
Middle	68	2	4	26	74	2	3	21
Lower	71	3	3	23	72	1	3	24
City Size								
Over 1 Million	57	3	5	35	61	3	6	30
100,000–1 Million	64	2	5	29	68	3	4	25
25,000–100,000	74	5	4	17	71	2	3	24
10,000–25,000	67	5	4	24	68	1	3	28
Under 10,000	76	2	3	19	77	2	2	19
Rural, farm	81	1	2	16	79	1	2	18

The question: *Do you think there is a Heaven, where people who have led good lives are eternally rewarded?*

(continued)

	1965				1952			
	BELIEVE IN AFTERLIFE			DON'T BELIEVE IN AFTERLIFE	BELIEVE IN AFTERLIFE			DON'T BELIEVE IN AFTERLIFE
	YES	NO	DON'T KNOW		YES	NO	DON'T KNOW	
	%	%	%	%	%	%	%	%
Region								
New England	58	4	5	33	74	1	3	22
Middle Atlantic	65	2	2	31	67	2	3	28
South Atlantic	76	2	2	20	79	1	2	18
East South Central	91	–	2	7	84	1	2	13
West South Central	78	1	1	20	85	1	1	13
East North Central	68	2	5	25	67	2	5	26
West North Central	71	1	8	20	74	2	3	21
Mountain	59	12	4	25	60	5	7	28
Pacific	51	6	8	35	67	5	4	24

The question: *Do you think there is a Hell, to which people who have led bad lives and die without being sorry are eternally damned?*

	1965				1952			
	BELIEVE IN AFTERLIFE			DON'T BELIEVE IN AFTERLIFE	BELIEVE IN AFTERLIFE			DON'T BELIEVE IN AFTERLIFE
	YES	NO	DON'T KNOW		YES	NO	DON'T KNOW	
	%	%	%	%	%	%	%	%
TOTAL	54	13	8	25	58	12	7	23
Religion								
Roman Catholic	70	7	6	17	74	5	6	15
Protestant total	54	15	9	22	56	15	9	20
Baptist	68	7	6	19	75	6	6	13
Methodist	44	17	14	25	51	15	11	23
Lutheran	49	22	7	22	59	11	8	22
Presbyterian	39	22	10	29	45	25	10	20
Episcopal	17	38	13	32	26	30	11	33
Congregational	25	37	3	35	35	17	11	37
Other denominations	63	13	7	17	52	18	8	22

The question: *Do you think there is a Hell, to which people who have led bad lives and die without being sorry are eternally damned?* (continued)

	1965				1952			
	BELIEVE IN AFTERLIFE			DON'T BELIEVE IN AFTERLIFE	BELIEVE IN AFTERLIFE			DON'T BELIEVE IN AFTERLIFE
	YES	NO	DON'T KNOW		YES	NO	DON'T KNOW	
	%	%	%	%	%	%	%	%
Jewish	3	9	5	83	15	12	8	65
Other and none	20	13	4	63	33	7	3	57
Sex								
Men	54	10	8	28	57	11	7	25
Women	55	15	7	23	59	13	8	20
Age								
18–24 years	56	13	4	27	59	9	7	25
25–34	54	13	7	26	58	11	7	24
35–44	55	11	7	27	59	11	7	23
45–54	51	13	9	27	54	14	8	24
55–64	56	13	7	24	58	14	8	20
65 & over	55	14	10	21	56	12	13	19
Race								
White	55	13	8	24	58	12	7	23
Nonwhite	47	6	8	39	64	7	8	21
Education								
0–8th grade	65	6	7	22	62	8	6	24
1–3 years high school	61	7	6	26	58	10	7	25
High school graduate	52	16	7	25	58	14	9	19
1–3 years college	47	20	10	23	50	17	11	22
College graduate	38	17	11	34	41	22	9	28
Occupation								
Professional	44	20	8	28	51	17	9	23
Proprietor or manager	51	18	8	23	52	15	7	26
White-collar worker	51	15	7	27	55	17	11	17
Service worker	60	4	8	28	62	10	8	20
Manual worker	58	10	7	25	61	9	6	24
Farmer	69	7	8	16	65	10	8	17
Nonlabor force	52	13	9	26	*	*	*	*

The question: *Do you think there is a Hell, to which people who have led bad lives and die without being sorry are eternally damned?* (continued)

	1965				1952			
	BELIEVE IN AFTERLIFE			DON'T BELIEVE IN AFTERLIFE	BELIEVE IN AFTERLIFE			DON'T BELIEVE IN AFTERLIFE
	YES	NO	DON'T KNOW		YES	NO	DON'T KNOW	
	%	%	%	%	%	%	%	%
Income								
Upper	44	19	10	27	50	17	10	23
Middle	55	12	7	26	57	14	8	21
Lower	59	10	8	23	63	6	7	24
City Size								
Over 1 Million	45	14	6	35	49	10	11	30
100,000–1 Million	48	14	9	29	52	14	9	25
25,000–100,000	62	13	8	17	62	8	6	24
10,000–25,000	55	15	6	24	50	15	7	28
Under 10,000	62	11	8	19	58	15	8	19
Rural, farm	69	7	8	16	72	6	4	18
Region								
New England	42	17	8	33	60	11	7	22
Middle Atlantic	53	12	4	31	50	15	7	28
South Atlantic	63	8	9	20	67	8	7	18
East South Central	85	2	6	7	77	6	4	13
West South Central	65	9	6	20	75	7	5	13
East North Central	54	14	7	25	52	11	11	26
West North Central	55	12	13	20	60	12	7	21
Mountain	34	27	14	25	35	30	7	28
Pacific	35	21	9	35	47	19	10	24

The question: *Do you think there is any real possibility of your going there?*

	1965				1952			
	BELIEVE IN HELL			DON'T BELIEVE IN HELL	BELIEVE IN HELL			DON'T BELIEVE IN HELL
	YES	NO	DON'T KNOW		YES	NO	DON'T KNOW	
	%	%	%	%	%	%	%	%
TOTAL	17	25	12	46	12	29	17	42
Religion								
Roman Catholic	27	23	20	30	20	26	28	26
Protestant total	15	29	11	45	12	32	12	44
Baptist	17	40	12	31	14	50	11	25
Methodist	10	23	11	56	11	28	12	49
Lutheran	17	24	8	51	10	31	18	41
Presbyterian	15	15	9	61	10	28	7	55
Episcopal	5	5	8	82	8	13	5	74
Congregational	5	12	8	75	11	15	9	65
Other denominations	19	32	11	38	12	26	14	48
Jewish	2	1	–	97	4	4	7	85
Other and none	6	7	7	80	10	8	15	67
Sex								
Men	20	21	13	46	14	25	18	43
Women	14	28	12	46	11	32	16	41
Age								
18–24 years	24	20	12	44	19	27	13	41
25–34	21	22	12	45	16	27	15	42
35–44	19	24	12	45	14	29	16	41
45–54	15	24	12	49	10	28	16	46
55–64	14	28	14	44	11	30	17	42
65 & over	9	33	13	45	9	33	14	44
Race								
White	18	25	13	44	15	27	16	42
Nonwhite	8	28	11	53	15	36	13	36
Education								
0–8th grade	13	35	17	35	11	31	20	38
1–3 years high school	19	27	14	40	14	28	16	42
High school graduate	18	23	11	48	16	27	15	42
1–3 years college	18	19	10	53	13	26	11	50
College graduate	17	15	6	62	8	24	9	59

The question: *Do you think there is any real possibility of your going there?* (continued)

	1965 BELIEVE IN HELL			DON'T BELIEVE IN HELL	1952 BELIEVE IN HELL			DON'T BELIEVE IN HELL
	YES	NO	DON'T KNOW		YES	NO	DON'T KNOW	
	%	%	%	%	%	%	%	%
Occupation								
Professional	18	19	7	56	12	28	11	49
Proprietor or manager	15	25	10	50	15	26	11	48
White-collar worker	19	21	11	49	12	27	16	45
Service worker	15	21	23	41	16	30	16	38
Manual worker	19	25	14	42	14	28	19	39
Farmer	20	35	14	31	12	34	19	35
Nonlabor force	11	31	11	47	*	*	*	*
Income								
Upper	17	19	8	56	10	29	11	50
Middle	17	24	13	46	14	26	17	43
Lower	16	30	14	40	16	28	19	37
City Size								
Over 1 Million	20	17	9	54	13	19	17	51
100,000–1 Million	16	22	10	52	12	24	16	48
25,000–100,000	13	30	19	38	16	21	25	38
10,000–25,000	16	24	15	45	18	17	15	50
Under 10,000	17	31	14	38	12	32	14	42
Rural, farm	16	35	17	32	17	40	15	28
Region								
New England	14	20	8	58	16	18	26	40
Middle Atlantic	19	20	14	47	11	18	21	50
South Atlantic	16	32	16	36	13	40	14	33
East South Central	32	43	10	15	21	45	11	23
West South Central	15	33	17	35	17	45	13	25
East North Central	16	25	13	46	11	26	15	48
West North Central	24	21	10	45	16	21	23	40
Mountain	10	18	7	65	3	22	10	65
Pacific	9	19	7	65	15	22	10	53

DESIGN OF THE GALLUP SAMPLE

The design of the sample used by the Gallup Poll for its standard surveys of public opinion is that of a replicated probability sample down to the block level in the case of urban areas and to segments of townships in the case of rural areas.

After stratifying the nation geographically and by size of community in order to insure conformity of the sample with the latest available estimates by the Census Bureau of the distribution of the adult population, over 350 different sampling locations or areas (Census Tracts or Census Enumeration Districts) are selected on a mathematically random basis from within cities, towns, and counties which have in turn been selected on a mathematically random basis. The interviewers have no choice whatsoever concerning the part of the city, town, or county in which they conduct their interviews.

Approximately five interviews are conducted in each such randomly selected sampling point. Interviewers are given maps of the area to which they are assigned, with a starting point indicated; they are required to follow a specified direction. At each occupied dwelling unit, interviewers are instructed to select respondents by following a prescribed systematic method and by a male-female assignment. This procedure is followed until the assigned number of interviews has been completed.

Since this sampling procedure is designed to produce a sample which approximates the adult civilian population (18 and older) living in private households in the United States (that is, excluding those in prisons and hospitals, hotels, religious and educational institutions, and on military reservations), the survey results can be applied to this population for the purpose of projecting percentages into number of people. The manner in which the sample is drawn also produces a sample which approximates the population

221

of private households in the United States. Therefore, survey results can also be projected in terms of number of households when appropriate.

Sampling Error

In interpreting survey results, it should be remembered that all sample surveys are subject to sampling error, that is, the extent to which the results may differ from what would be obtained if the whole population surveyed had been interviewed. The size of such sampling errors depends largely on the number of interviews.

In the interest of readability we have referred throughout this book to survey estimates as if they were "true" values. In fact, all figures derived from sample surveys are estimates, and, as such, subject to error.

The sample base for most of the surveys of the general public reported in this book are based on in-person interviews with a minimum of 1500 adults, 18 and older, interviewed in more than 300 scientifically selected localities across the nation. For results based on samples of this size, one can say with 95 percent confidence that the error attributable to sampling and other random effects, in terms of the *national* findings, could be three percentage points in either direction.

Projections

When projections have been made from estimates of proportions to numbers of persons, we have referred in each case to some fixed number of persons. A more technical presentation might offer not just a projected number of persons, but a number accompanied by a range reflecting the fact that the basis for the projection is an estimate.

Index